Health and Medicine
in the Reformed Tradition

Health/Medicine and the Faith Traditions

Edited by Martin E. Marty and Kenneth L. Vaux

Health/Medicine and the Faith Traditions
explores the ways in which major religions
relate to the questions of human well-being.
It issues from Project Ten,
an international program of the
Lutheran General Medical Center
in Park Ridge, Illinois.

Health and Medicine in the Reformed Tradition

PROMISE, PROVIDENCE,
AND CARE

Kenneth L. Vaux

Crossroad · New York

1984
The Crossroad Publishing Company
370 Lexington Avenue, New York, N.Y. 10017

Library of Congress Cataloging in Publication Data

Vaux, Kenneth.
Health and medicine in the reformed tradition.
Includes bibliographical references.
1. Health—Religious aspects—Reformed Church—History
of doctrines. 2. Medicine—Religious aspects—Reformed
Church—History of doctrines. 3. Reformed Church—
Doctrines—History. 4. Health—Religious aspects—
Presbyterian Church—History of doctrines. 5. Medicine—
Religious aspects—Presbyterian Church—History of
doctrines. 6. Presbyterian Church—Doctrines—History.
I. Title.
BX9423.H43V38   1983   261.5'6   83-15295
ISBN 0-8245-0612-X

Contents

Foreword

"Health" we know and "Medicine" we know, but what is the "Reformed Tradition"? Since health and medicine come to us in part through institutions—hospitals, clinics, pharmacies, and the like—and since they can become corrupt and malformed, it would be natural to think that Kenneth Vaux is talking about the reform of such institutions. What he has to say may have a bearing on that kind of reform. Yet it is not what he has in mind first of all.

This book belongs to a series on Health/Medicine and the *Faith* Traditions. There. It is out. The subject is religion. That should be enough to repel many people who would have read on had it to do only with clinics and hospitals. At the very least, many could ignore it. They have other things to do than to see what faith traditions have to say about health, or what medicine has to say about religion. To such potential readers I wish I could reach out and say, "Read on, no matter what preconceptions you bring to the book."

Why? Because the author and those he has inspired to work with him on the Faith Traditions project have a thesis to propose. If the thesis as a whole is supportable, its workings out can have a bearing on human good. That ought to interest anyone who cares about the well being of others or, for that matter, anyone who cares about his or her own health and wholeness.

The project commends historians to survey the long history of religious traditions, be they Hindu, Buddhist, Muslim, Jewish, Christian, or "none of the above." They simply need to be living traditions, which shape and are shaped by people of our time. Out of these surveys the historians dredge the motifs which concentrate on health and medicine. Alongside this company of scholars are representatives of the traditions who can speak out of them, to them, in some ways for them. In still another phase of the project the theses of these companies and representatives will be tested in clinics or home situations. The present book represents the "representative" tradition.

Now we are ready to talk about the Reformed Tradition, and why anyone in it—which means several million Americans and millions elsewhere—

and, more, why anyone outside it should care. The *Oxford English Diction-ary* notes that Reformed "sometimes include all the Protestant churches," and continues, appropriately for Professor Vaux's book, "and sometimes [the term] is specifically restricted to the Calvinistic bodies as contrasted with the Lutheran." That Vaux was supposed to keep his hands off the Lutheran tradition, which he more or less does, is clear from the fact that as his partner in the project I have just written on Lutheranism. That he cannot have all the rest of Protestantism to himself is clear from the fact that, well under way, are books on the Anglican, Methodist, "evangelical," and other Protestant heritages.

We still have some way to go to locate the work. The *World Christian Encyclopedia*, edited by David B. Barrett (Oxford, 1982), estimates that three years after publication, in 1985, there will be 39,283,735 "affiliated" people in global Reformed Christianity, alongside 43,539,026 Lutherans in their pure form. Yet in much of Europe the Reformed and Lutherans do not strain their traditions so purely, which is why Vaux can only "more or less" stay away from my Lutheran turf. Reformed and Lutherans "united," according to the encyclopedia, total 65,163,979 people. If the project advisors and publishers can attract the notice of a tiny percentage of these millions, the book can serve their enormous house well.

Assuming that some Reformed and "united" Protestants may ignore the help this book can give them, let me try to pick up a market or, in scholarly terms, indicate the relevance of this work, for others. Boldly and baldly let me put it this way: *modern* medical care, hospitals, clinics, and medical technology grew up in large part on the territory shaped by what we may call semi-secularized Reformed Protestantism. Vaux's homelands include Switzerland, the Netherlands, France, much of Germany, Scotland, most of North America through Reformed Puritan influence, and wherever else the heirs of reformer John Calvin and his colleagues gave shape to the spiritual life of the Protestant world. (England should also belong to this map, especially because of the Puritan influence, but official religion in England is Anglican, and that will receive a separate book.)

We can put a fine edge on things and say that the inventors, discoverers, and builders of technological medicine did not wake up in the morning seeing how they could apply the teachings of Jesus as mediated through John Calvin to the healing of others. This company included citizens who never were Christian or Protestant or Reformed, along with others who had drifted away and opposed or ignored the traditions. Many inside it may have never thought about connecting their religion and their research or health care. Millions of nonprofessionals who were members may have put "religion" in one box and "health" in another.

All that may be true, but it still does not lessen the urgency of exploring how what is in the two boxes connects. The hospital and health traditions we have, and which were exported to much of the world by medical, religious, and technological missionaries, may have come from a "post-Protestant" world. That world, however, is much different that it would have been had it been post-Buddhist, post-Hindu, post-Muslim, or whatever. Much of our life and thought is reflexive, instinctive, involuntary, and healers on Reformed soil carry with them certain assumptions about life which they would otherwise not carry. It is time to examine these.

This is precisely what Kenneth Vaux does. What does it mean that the ancestors of these millions of people, a creative lot, saw themselves as "elect" and God as "sovereign"? What difference does it make that they developed such a strong sense of a "calling" that when Puritans turned Yankee or Protestants turned capitalist, they were almost compulsive about seeing that the Protestant ethic remained a work ethic, and what does all that have to do with health today? Reformed Christians believe that they are to be stewards in special ways of their bodies, their cultures, and these ways affect others who never heard of John Calvin or never entered a Presbyterian church.

I do not want to anticipate the contents of this book any further, or to intrude on the territory Kenneth Vaux knows and expounds so well. I only want to say that I am a bit envious of the company he gets to keep. In theology he can drop names and pick up themes from John Calvin, John Knox, the founder of modern theology Friedrich Schleiermacher, the twentieth-century giant Karl Barth, the greatest American religious thinker Jonathan Edwards, modern psychiatrist Karl Menninger, and political theologian Jürgen Moltmann. If you need theological brains to pick, this is awesome company. They are not household or hospitalhold names, of course. Showing how and why they might be, or how and why their thought can help people who never knew their names and may never read a page of their works, is the task of Kenneth Vaux. Whoever gives him a patient hour or two will find that he does this with a sense of at-homeness in the Reformed tradition. He couples this with a concern that we at least visit that "home," profit from its environment, and carry some of its products and ethos to the surrounding world. Because Vaux is so at home and because he treats his subject profoundly and with a concern for contemporary application, I assure that all readers will become better informed and can find new ideas and instruments for the theme of "well-being."

MARTIN E. MARTY
The University of Chicago

Preface

It is thought that people make moral decisions in two ways. In the first style of moral reasoning persons or groups move from basic principles to axioms about behavior to specific actions. But persons also make decisions on the basis of what they believe about God, themselves, and the universe. In what we might call faith reasoning, where one deals with profound moral questions such as those involving life and death, persons move from belief to values to concrete imperatives for action. This work studies the latter mode of moral decision making, that approach called theological ethics.

The purpose of this study is twofold. Beginning with the premise that our moral life is shaped by that faith tradition in which we stand, it sets out first to probe the tenets of one such tradition, the Protestant Reformed (also called Calvinist or Presbyterian). What makes this tradition unique? What is its understanding of the nature of God? Second, the study asks: How does man respond to God and to other human persons? That is, how do theological perceptions shape ethical behaviors? Briefly stated, the Reformed tradition has contended, and does contend, that ethics must be defined with reference first to God, who is the source of goodness and purpose in the world, and, second, with reference to other persons, who are morally conflicted beings capable of both good and evil. Karl Barth, the great modern Reformed theologian, has spoken of human existence itself as being the theme of the Word of God: that is, our knowledge of God and our service of him are inextricably intertwined.[1] This presupposition that God's nature determines our nature, that God's life animates our life, and that his love and justice direct our ethics, has undergirded Reformed ethics from the sixteenth century on to our day.

But to acknowledge the interrelation of beliefs and values, even to fully analyze the rich heritage in which beliefs and values have their life, is not adequate. Theological reasoning and historical analysis awaken and enlighten, but in this study these will be used also as tools for decision making.

We will move constantly from the past to the present, from the given to the possible, from the resolved to the troubling, as we explore the bearing of the Reformed faith tradition on our experiences of health and disease. Theology in the Reformed understanding concerns not only God's overarching purpose in redeeming the cosmos—the divine drama—but the human pilgrimage from birth to death. Sacred history (*Heilsgeschichte*) continually intersects with human history (*Lebensgeschichte*) as we live out our daily lives. God acts; we respond, as Luther has said. Whether we respond creatively or destructively affects all aspects of our life, as choices—both perennial ones and new ones created by our technologically sophisticated world—are thrust upon us.

I am a Presbyterian. My family upbringing, church experience, and higher education have all been shaped by that tradition. My ancestors were German Reformed and Scots-Irish Presbyterian immigrants to the United States. I have been nurtured in the faith brought to Scotland from Geneva by John Knox; the teaching of the German-Reformed movement expressed in the Heidelberg Catechism; the theology of the English Puritans under the Stuarts and Parliament, and the transmission of this doctrine by the Dutch and Scots and Scots-Irish Calvinists and the persecuted pilgrims who came to the New World, the place George III woefully called "that Presbyterian Commonwealth." This study of the Reformed tradition's understanding of health and disease could have been written by a Czech, Swiss, or French Reformed Protestant, or by someone whose background has been one of the sectarian Calvinist movements that flourished in Europe and America beginning in the seventeenth century. My perspective is but one shaft of light from the Calvinist prism, which itself is a singular beam from the multifaceted jewel of Judeo-Christian truth.

Calvinism is a dynamic tradition, always changing, adapting to and creating a new ethos. It may be expressed in the political witness of Mayor Jacques Ellul of Bordeaux, France, or of Bill Hudnut of Indianapolis, or in Scottish burial customs, or in political protest in Seoul, South Korea. In the Reformed tradition all areas of one's life properly belong to God: thus, all activities, including politics, can be seen as one's Christian vocation. This is *reformatio perennis*, an ongoing renewal. It seeks not only to interpret but to fashion continually a fresh and relevant biomedical ethos.

Some may puzzle over the value of exploring individual traditions in depth during a time when all persons of goodwill need to pool their forces if the earth is to survive. George Caldwell, president of our sponsoring medical center, has noted that in-depth studies of individual traditions, all concerned for problems of health and disease, will ultimately reveal a broad and deep common commitment to the human enterprise—will indeed accent rather than blunt the basic values we share. And those of us who believe that God is working out his purposes in human history suggest that the diversity in religious traditions that we have seen in recent centuries may be a necessary elaboration of a multifaceted truth which must occur as a prelude to a future symphony in which, in fact as in will, we again will be united.

I thank my partner in life and in this project, Sara Anson Vaux, who is in fact coauthor of this book, and our Riverside neighbor and friend Martin Marty, whose life story and scholarly pilgrimage have crossed paths with ours these recent years, bringing wisdom to Project X, the enterprise that gave rise to this book. Project X, administered by our able colleague David Stein, is an undertaking of the Lutheran General Medical Center in Chicago, one of the fine teaching centers related to the University of Illinois Health Center. This project has been designed to assemble, assess, and apply the theological wisdom of the world's great faith traditions to the questions of health and disease. This volume is organized around the ten themes of Project X and the helpful recasting of these themes offered by another colleague in the project, Dean Frank Sherman of the Lutheran School of Theology in Chicago.

Unless otherwise noted, all biblical references in this book are to the New English Bible.

KENNETH VAUX
Oxford

Introduction: Definitions

A crisis is some moment, some situation, that sweeps away routine and predictability, brings our life to a halt, and forces us consciously to choose and to act. The burden that our technological sophistication lays upon our sanity, our free will, even our very survival has made the grounds out of which such choices might be made a matter of searching interest. How are such choices (personal, political, technological) made? From what range of possible "goods" do we select one course of action? What factors determine our selection?

This book contends that, although our moral lives may be shaped by a host of factors (our genetic makeup; our family background; our ethnic or national identity; and, now, mass media), our religious beliefs—and the "faith tradition" within which we hold these beliefs—exert a powerful influence in determining how we will act at a time of crisis. From belief arises value, or priority; and out of priority issue our moral acts, consciously chosen.

The skeptic may well ask whether science, law, or philosophy might equally provide a system of universal ethics as valid as that transmitted by a faith tradition. Alasdair MacIntyre has argued persuasively, however, that our only viable ethical resources are those specific cultural manifestations we term historic faith traditions, which assemble, appropriate, and transmit to succeeding generations the experiences of a given believing and valuing community. Virtues, defined as ethical powers for living, can be possessed only as "part of a tradition in which we inherit them" and understand them.[1]

It is not the belief alone, then, that shapes the moral life of the believer but the combined power of historical inheritance and the presence of a faith community—other believers against whom one's beliefs and actions are continually being measured and tested and to whom one looks for dialogue and support. (I credit Martin E. Marty for this distinction.) Yet within the context of that shaping tradition, MacIntyre notes, "one's personal narrative is

1

both free and unique"[2] and as such interrelated with other narratives. That is, a person both receives his moral identity from, and contributes character to, a tradition. "Tradition," then, is a collective and historical concept within which the individual lives out his own history, his personal narrative of fears, hopes, and deeds—his "virtue." He draws strength from the tradition, but he also creates it by these acts. Thus virtue can be said to be both that system of ethical priorities which one comprehends through the tradition and those individual moral choices which one makes in the still, cold moments of personal crisis.

In discussing the effect that religious tradition exerts on decisions concerning health and disease, then, are we analyzing historical problems (past situations in which the actions of certain persons have been influenced clearly by their beliefs) or setting forth prescriptive modes (clearly defined aspects of one tradition that might serve as guidelines for contemporary persons seeking help in making terrible choices)? We do both, for in matters of health and disease we act both preventively and interventively. Tradition, both as that culmination of events and statements to which we consciously or unconsciously ascribe and as that wellspring of articulated wisdom from which we draw refreshment, determines how we act.

The "tradition" (in this case, "Reformed") possesses a number of clearly identifiable characteristics, basic underlying premises that set it apart from other traditions and shape the fundamental values of its adherents. Yet merely to list these characteristics would not do, for the Reformed tradition, like all traditions, emerged from some aspects of preexisting traditions that must be credited to some extent with formulating our world view. In no age have believers lived in a glass case: no tradition has remained impervious to cultural and historical influence. The Reformed faith certainly shares much with other Protestant traditions, with modern Catholicism, and with Judaism. History continually impinges upon tradition: the past shapes the present. And it is in the present that we are making new choices: in crisis looking back at the past to draw from it strength, and help, and perhaps enough vision to enable us to endure this present time.

Traditions, then, are dynamic and therefore elusive. "Like a canal reef," Gordon Rupp has said, traditions consist of millions of tiny cells, "in this case the lives of millions of humble, believing men and women."[3] If the Reformed tradition is as flexible and various as the number of its believers—furthermore, if its most recognizable proponents acknowledge that it does but "sustain" the "catholic substance" of Christianity, as Tillich argued (which in turn implies a strong paternal link with Judaism and with Eastern religions)—wherein lies its originality, its claim to be other than a universal system of general beliefs about our universe? The answer will be found, of course, in examining the statements of beliefs and the specific actions of believers. To state that the Reformers saw man's relationship with God and the human task in the world in a fresh way is not to deny any debt to history: indeed, the Reformers saw themselves as "conservative" or "restorative," hearkening back to the church fathers, the primitive church, the Bible, and the Hebrew covenant for correctives to what they saw as distortions in belief raised by the medieval Aristotelian synthesis of Aquinas and the Roman Catholic church.

In defining the nature of tradition, MacIntyre wrote that the present both responds to and comments upon the past, recognizing that its present interpretation of reality may in turn be "corrected and transcended by some yet more adequate future point of view."[4] That this has been and is true of the Reformed tradition we have noted, for in its very nature it is consciously both conservative (that is, radical, grateful for its "roots") and contemporary. But all modern faith traditions must acknowledge some common historical sources. How selections and corrections were made becomes a matter of major concern when differing interpretations of reality are brought to bear upon a specific current medical problem, for instance. Points of difference cannot be analyzed until these pools of commonality have been credited.

In the covenant of life initiated by Yahweh with the people of Israel in the late second millennium B.C., the Reformed tradition has found its earliest ethical grounding. From this point onward, all of life's experiences and decisions were to be seen in the light of God's will for his human creation. Moral acts did not, do not, exist in a cosmic vacuum, but are relational: tied to a God who could be known and implored, and through him, to other humans. Human accountability—the sense of being held responsible for our acts— was founded in a covenant that embraced all facets of existence.

The Reformers looked, then, to the Noachian law, pre-Sinai (pre-Mosaic) teaching in Israel. They studied anew the law and the prophets. They returned to the primitive Christian communities, fellowships of persons who "turned the world upside down," who lived and died not unto themselves but unto Christ, and saw their life's purpose as facilitating God's unfolding redemptive project in the world. They scrutinized the writings of Saint Augustine. They were touched by the words and witness of Jan Hus, John Wycliffe, Peter Waldo and others who preceded them. Their standpoint was both self-consciously historical, reflecting on its heritage, but also self-consciously dynamic, vital, and contemporary, seeking to articulate a fresh witness for a needy time.

In this context, who were these "Reformers," the seminal thinkers in our uniquely Reformed heritage? They were John Calvin and the Geneva reformers, and John Knox and the authors of the Scots Confession of 1560. Our modern Reformed tradition embraces them with their interpretations of past faith traditions but has also looked to the continuing revelations interpreted by English Puritans, such as John Milton and Thomas Sydenham; to American Puritans such as Cotton Mather and Jonathan Edwards; to sermons, hymns, polity, and liturgy from the sixteenth to the twentieth centuries, and to Friedrich Schleiermacher, F. D. Maurice and Karl Barth. Who are the Reformers of today? All those who claim kinship with this long tradition.

Some thinkers, like Arnold Toynbee, have seen Reformed belief and its derivative ethical system as something quite striking, even miraculous. During the two centuries following 1563, Toynbee argued, Western civilization took greater strides forward than it had done since the Roman Empire. How does Toynbee define this "progress"? First, Western thinkers challenged their traditions, heritage, and "inherited doctrines" by "examining the phenomena independently" and by doing "their own thinking." They now chose to coexist "peacefully with heterodox minorities, no longer feeling an obligation . . . to impose a majority's creed and rite by force."[5]

Weber and Tawney pinpointed the Protestant spirit as what they believed to be a unique understanding of human dealing in this world under God: an understanding that fashioned a distinctive ethos, in this case, the drive to control, to excel.[6] The proportion of Protestants, particularly Calvinists, among prominent businessmen, scholars, and scientists is indeed striking: does the ethos propel the drive, or does a person of that temperament gravitate toward a tradition that recognizes, even applauds, the positive exercise of human will? Certainly, as V. H. H. Green has noted, Protestant teaching promoted a life-style—sober, hard-working, honest, virtuous—that fostered action and trust.[7]

Other historians would question the broad sweep of such an analysis, protesting first that such intellectual "independence" and spiritual "tolerance" were well-prepared for during earlier ages; conversely, again, that the Reformation was "the last of the great medieval movements" (V. H. H. Green) or that such intellectual liberation waited for the Enlightenment. Second, detractors remind us that Reformers were zealous, sometimes bloody, in advancing their own causes: Calvin joined the persecutions of Michael Servetus, Oliver Cromwell, that of the Roman Catholics and the Quakers. Here is further evidence that toleration awaited the Enlightenment.[8] Nonetheless, Cromwell's well-known comment "Think it not impossible you might be wrong" and his lifting of censorship strike for the modern reader a new and much-welcome note of open-mindedness.

Historical wonder or parasite? Innovation or radical departure? The faith traditions fired during these centuries of blood and change did nonetheless accent both freedom and toleration against a time-locked ecclesiastical and political status quo. That both seminal thinkers and neophytes valued protest, question, and inquiry appears in the very name tagged onto them en masse: "Protestant." Reformation faiths were therefore both purist and humanist: that is, they sought to renovate historic truth (the long string of "traditions" from which they sprang) in the light of new knowledge. God and man were partners: moral law, originating with God, encircled human action, yet man acted creatively in freedom. God was sovereign and mankind sinful, yet human life had been gloriously redeemed through Christ. The moral life was grounded in the written Word, the Scriptures, and in the Living Word, Christ, as it was unfolded through preaching, literature, art, political and communal life, and personal relationships. Thus was God glorified, not blasphemed, through human creativity in science, work, and politics, for believers were seen as stewards over God's good gifts of mind and will. In all of life's events God's blessing and providence was to be seen. Man was thus not fettered, but constrained and guided, in his pursuit of truth. The change in perspective was to prove crucial: seen in this light, human energies were no longer diabolical but heavenly, joined in partnership with God in the mastery over creation.

> When I look up at the heavens, the work of thy fingers
>   the moon and the stars set in their place,
> what is man that thou shouldst remember him,
>   mortal man that thou shouldst care for him?
> Yet thou hast made him little less than a god,
>   crowning him with glory and honor.
> Thou makest him master over all thy creatures;
>   thou hast put everything under his feet....
> O Lord our sovereign,
>   how glorious is thy name in all the world! (Ps. 8)

Part I

WHAT DO
WE BELIEVE?
THE NATURE
OF GOD

I believe in God the Father Almighty, maker of heaven and earth, and in Jesus Christ, his only son our Lord.... (Apostles Creed)

How does the Reformed tradition envisage the nature of God? And God being so understood, how does man respond? Because of these beliefs and that relationship, how do we contour our lives not only to confront crisis but to live in joy and freedom? What pictures of the ultimate, of human nature and destiny, can guide us in the challenge of life and death?

Reformed belief about God and his creation can be presented in many formats, here under "creative sovereignty," "reconciliation," and "redemption." Briefly stated, God, though all-powerful, continually creates and recreates us as he works out his overarching purposes. Mankind, though often rebellious rather than receptive to God's will, is his partner in this ongoing process. Reformed theology contends that God's creative sovereignty invites humans from self-will to stewardship. God's reconciling purpose invites us no longer to impede, but rather be instrumental to, his work. The unity of creation and redemption in the ongoing work of God invites us to abandon our own schemes of salvation and to receive instead his new creation.

The Reformed tradition, and Reformed theology generally, is (as has been said earlier) multiform, as its peoples have touched and been touched by the great intellectual movements of the centuries. On the three topics here suggested (sovereignty, reconciliation, redemption), however, the biblical basis of Reformed theology has guarded a central core of thinking that sets it apart from other interpretations of the human situation. Perhaps the best way to encapsule Reformed belief is to look to one of the great statesmen of this faith tradition, the American Presbyterian John Mackay, who was educated in Scotland and at Princeton, and served as a missionary in Spain and South America before beginning a distinguished twenty-five-year presidency at Princeton Theological Seminary.

For Mackay, the essence of Calvinism lies in human obedience to the truth of God.[1] Like Luther, John Calvin was overwhelmed by the merciful grace of God. Whereas Luther stressed the subjective, personal side of Christianity (which gave rise to his matchless sermons and hymns), Calvin accented the objective reality of the sovereign God. Similarly, whereas Luther stressed justification by faith and the intrapsychic dynamics of guilt and forgiveness, Calvin favored the absoluteness and supremacy of the will of God in the history of the world and the destiny of human persons. Calvin's hymn of praise to God, the burning devotion of his heart, was expressed in his great theological treatise *The Institutes of the Christian Religion.*[2] This book expounds the truth of God and his sovereign purpose for mankind and the universe.

Just as the twentieth-century Reformed theologian Thomas Torrance has woven scientific insights from modern physics and cosmology together with theological wisdom into what he calls a theology of light, so Calvin in the *Institutes* drew together the scientific wisdom of his time into a systematic theological treatise. The heart of Calvin's doctrine is God's sovereign rule over nature, history, and all things human. When the Calvinists in Scotland, Holland, Switzerland, or America looked for devotion, they, like Calvin himself, turned to the Psalms. Here in the sublime poetry of David they found extolled "the God of the whole earth," who reigns over the creation, guiding it into its fulfillment and toward its consummation. Human destiny is also embraced in this sovereignty: "the Lord is the stronghold of my life; of whom shall I be afraid?"

The subsidiary doctrine that bears most directly on our study of the theology of human life and death is the doctrine of predestination and election. As God has guided the history of his chosen people through triumphs and crises, so he guides the destiny of the human race in the providence of his will. He undergirds our life as creative sovereign, reconciles us with himself and with one another, and continues to redeem our troubled existence as we struggle with what we are and what we are growing to be.

·1·

The Reformed Tradition:
Beliefs and Questions

CREATIVE SOVEREIGNTY

In his lifelong project, *Church Dogmatics*, Karl Barth articulated a latter-day Reformed position on the nature of God and his creation. Barth rejected the notions that the existence of God is self-evident and that man is by nature *homo religiosus*. For Barth, as for the Reformed tradition, we would know of no God were it not for his speech, his expression. God's creative sovereignty is conveyed in his communication. This is the subject of Parts I and II of the *Dogmatics*: "Word of God" and "God." It is only the breakthrough of Christ into time and space through his life, death, and resurrection that confirms to the world the history of Israel's covenant and the story of salvation.

The cornerstone of theology is that "God is." God has given himself to us to be known. This knowledge is also knowledge about ourselves and the movements and meanings of our life.

> We confess and acknowledge this our God to have created man, to wit, our first father Adam, to our own image and similitude, to whom he gave wisdom, Lordship, justice, free-will and clear knowledge of himself. . . .[1]

If the doctrine of the revelation of God tells us something of who God is and, therefore, who we are, the doctrine of God tells of God's activity and who we are becoming. God acts in the realm of nature. Who we are becoming, the passage of our life, is, in this sense, a divine activity. The poet has said: "Our times are in his hands." Therefore, events—what happens to us and what we make happen—are morally formed before God.

God is the guardian of our life's transitions. "The Lord will guard your going and your coming now and evermore" (Ps. 121:8).

> The sun rises and the sun goes down; back it returns to its place and rises there again. The wind blows south, the wind blows north, round and round it goes and returns full circle. All streams run into the sea, yet the sea never overflows; back to the place from which the streams ran they return to run again. . . . For everything its season and for every activity under heaven its time. (Eccl. 1:5–7, 3:1)

Though in one sense the Preacher intones a lament about the futility of all, he also believes that God is in and about nature's events: sun, wind, rain, seasons. Therefore, our fallings and risings, our comings and goings, not only awake God's interest and surveillance but also constitute the reality of his movements.

God is not just God in the abstract. God is God for us. God is the father of Jesus Christ, the man, made Lord. God without Jesus Christ, said Barth, does not exist. Therefore, God is known only as the "maker of the covenant between Himself and Man" (*Dogmatics*, II/2, p. 509). The substance of the covenant is the moral command undergirded by the relational promise. The essence of the Old Testament is that God will be God to those who follow his will. Jesus echoed: "If anyone wills to do my will he will know the source of my teaching" (John 7:17). While the will of God for some may contain secret revelations of the divine or glimpses into the future, its essence is conveyed in the ethical requirement. God knows us and chooses us to be of service, to join him in his work. God is present to us in Gospel and in law. Law in this sense is the Word of God: the Torah and prophets, the Gospel lessons, the instruction of the apostles. Ethics, summarized Barth, "belongs to the doctrine of God" (*Dogmatics*, II/2, p. 512).

God is; man is becoming. The Apostles Creed embraces this intertwining of gift and response. Luther recognized it in referring to the *Gabe* and the *Aufgabe*. Barth develops the dialectic of divine action and human response throughout the *Dogmatics*. The Reformed tradition recognizes realistically the ambivalent and paradoxical nature of our inclinations: to God's good gift of himself we may be receptive or rebellious, facilitating or frustrating his plans for human history, for our own lives. The general bent of a life as it passes through time may lean toward either the creative or the negative, as Erik Erikson has illustrated, but yet tension remains throughout. Perhaps the conflict between life-affirming and life-denying forces was fairly accurately portrayed by the good and evil angels who struggled for Faustus's soul. The Reformed tradition acknowledges this duality in the human nature that responds to God's perfection. It recognizes further the ambiguous and elusive landscape in which moral choices characteristically are made.

In the beginning of creation, when God made heaven and earth, the earth was without form and void, and darkness over the face of the abyss, and a mightly wind that swept over the surface of the waters. God said, "Let there be light," and there was light . . . . (Gen. 1:1–2)

When all things began, the Word already was. The Word dwelt with God, and what God was, the Word was. The Word, then, was with God at the beginning, and through him all things came to be; no single thing was created without him. All that came to be was alive with his life, and that life was the light of men. (John 1:1–4)

God's creative sovereignty comes to abide with our life in his incarnate truth, which the early Christians described as Logos, meaning word, person, and wisdom. God has known us, thereby making self-knowledge possible. Our health thus must be measured against that awesome yet loving ideal, the God known to us through Christ, the living Word. What we understand of that revelation (that is, what we conceive to be the nature of God and what implications this understanding carries for our relations with other persons) thus determines our posture, not only in healing disease but also in nurturing well-being.

The earliest philosophers and theologians, seeking to capture some picture of the "ideal man," often recognized that a divine force hovered around human persons. Plato, for instance, spoke of a divine grounding for all reality, an ultimate realm of which persons as well as phenomena were but pale reflections. Spirit penetrated matter and personality.

The Hebrews, building upon Oriental cultures in which a transcending, divine presence had been acknowledged, conceived of this presence, Yahweh, as a God who was Word: that is, he made his will known through law and the prophets. He *revealed* himself to his chosen people. That revelation crystallized (after centuries of debate) around A.D. 100, when the Jewish Synod identified a set sacred literature, a group of books accepted as unfolding the holy story of God as he guided his people.

The spoken and written word became living Word as Word became flesh in Jesus Christ, who for believers personified the Hebrew will and word of God. As Melito of Sardis phrased this belief, "The law became word and the old became new . . . . The command became grace" (ca. A.D. 170).[2] To the Hellenistic mind this Jesus was the historical revelation of Logos, that principle which the Greeks felt provided the rationale of the entire universe. The preaching and teaching of the primitive Christian community along with its apostolic correspondence was added to the Old Testament canon to form the Christian written word, the Gospels, the Epistles, and the Revelation of the New Testament. Although occasionally in Christian history new revelation has been claimed and in some traditions subsequent dogma has been promulgated, the Christian tradition in general has seen the apostolic age as culminating verbal and historic revelation.

In the Reformed tradition, then, the Word (revelation) necessarily precedes any other discussion of the attributes of the nature of God, for it is through revelation that this nature is known. Further, in Reformed thought, knowledge and service, God and his world, are inextricably linked: all the world was meant to be and what it is becoming is disclosed in Christ, the Word. "In Christ," Tillich wrote, "eschatology is fulfilled and a new reality has started."[3] Within the wide range of interpretations about what this "cosmic Christology" might be, C. F. D. Moule perhaps expresses the normative center of the Reformed tradition in finding the heart of Christian truth in the "ultimacy" of Christ as revealed in Colossians, Hebrews, and John.[4] Hebrews opens thus:

> When in former times God spoke to our forefathers, he spoke in fragmentary and varied fashion through the prophets. But in this the final age he has spoken to us in the Son whom he has made heir to the whole universe, and through whom he created all orders of existence. The Son who is the effulgence of God's splendor and the stamp of God's very being, and sustains the universe by his word of power. (Heb. 1:1–3)

Christ is the mediator of a "new covenant," one which embraces the whole world of human experience.

The cosmos coheres through Christ, the revealed Word. In the words of our earliest creed, he is the one "through whom everything is."[5]

> [Christ] is the image of the invisible God; his is the primacy over all created things. In him everything in heaven and on earth was created . . . the whole universe has been created through him and for him. And he exists before everything, and all things are held together in him. (Col. 1:15–17)

God through Christ has revealed himself, then, as the creator and ruler of the cosmos. In him is our health and our salvation. But in Reformed thought the divine-human relationship is one of partnership rather than respectful distance, perhaps most accurately visualized in Michelangelo's fresco of the Creation story on the Sistine Chapel ceiling: God reaches out to touch mankind with his energizing power. The Reformed tradition in the spirit of Calvin is a "worldly" tradition, loving the earth, taking the world and the human body very seriously, not only because of Christ's incarnation but because Christ lies at the very heart of all reality. As Einstein once commented to Tillich, the divine (Logos) is the miracle of the structure of reality.[6] Such a world view shapes the Christian's moral life, for each experience and each opportunity reflects the eschatological reality of Christ. The Christian asks, "What is being done in this world through Christ? How do I understand 'what is' (nature) and 'what is happening' (history) in the light of that center?" These questions affect relationships, politics, science—all areas of life. In science, for instance, the unfolding of genetic knowledge as well as moral decisions about genetic engineering refer to this central understanding of the cosmos—that it belongs to God through Christ.

That same Christ shows us what it is to be fully human. Before a provident God and within a resplendent world we find ourselves both known and loved: we know and love in response. Our minds discern in nature an order that works: nature's laws, cause and effect, memory, analytical reason, anticipation. These abilities create all science, technology, and art. Reason is the endowment that allows us to comprehend nature's constitution and its movement. We know (reason) because we are known by God, that ultimate reality bound by neither space nor time.

Compassion, or agape love, like knowledge, is a grace, not an instinct— a grace bestowed on man in the image of God. Animals display affinity within and between species, but that only ensures survival. Humans are capable of feeling connected with and concerned about others; they are not compelled to be just and caring, but rather sense that they achieve their identity through reciprocity. Such qualities flow from God in Christ. Receptivity to Christ's spirit "arouses others to love and active goodness." A compassionate, peaceful, and virtuous life, Paul counseled the Hebrews, shows the Lord to the world (Heb. 12:14).

Health, then, might be defined as that state of being in which we fully embody the image of God, for God through Christ has shown us our true self—what we are meant to be. But health in this sense has always been lost; as the old Book of Common Prayer intoned, "There is no health in us."

> When the Lord saw that man had done much evil on earth and that his thoughts and inclinations were always evil, he was sorry that he had made man on earth, and he was grieved at heart. (Gen. 6:5)

The great burden of ruin is inflicted by our knowing and willing selves. Knowledge of the good, the "ought," the ideal of "health," seems to bear no causal relation to doing the good, as Paul succinctly articulated:

> The good which I *want* to do, I fail to do; but what I do is the wrong which is against my will; and if what I do is against my will, clearly it is no longer I who am the agent, but sin that has its lodging in me. (Rom. 7:19–20)

Unfortunately, the gifts of reason and compassion with which we have been endowed as tools for serving God through exploring the cosmos and caring for each other can damn as well as save. Theology refers to this ongoing anthropological crisis as the Fall. Knowledge itself is seductive. The road to greater and greater promise is the same road into great danger. The knowledge and utilization of mechanical energy, electrical energy, then nuclear energy, for example, represents a progression into greater power and therefore greater responsibility. Similarly, the movement from knowing and controlling human movements to depth psychology to DNA deciphering is, as Goethe might have put it, a journey into the unknown, the unpredictable, the treacherous. When we speak of the secrets or mysteries of nature, of the "forbidden experiment" or of "playing God," we are acknowledging zones which cause pause as the mind crosses the frontier from known to unknown.

But all health has not been denied us: we retain just enough of the "good nature" of our original creation "whereby to wail the loss of the rest," as Augustine has said. "Yet does not God . . . punish the good which he himself created, but the evil which the devil committed," "the devil" here symbolizing not so much an external malevolent force but our own rebellion against who God means us to be and how we are to relate to those around us.[7] We honor God's name as we give our life over to him and live by his rule in our life's decisions. His creative sovereignty is the standard and sustenance of our life.

RECONCILIATION

God has revealed himself through Christ as creative, sovereign ruler of the cosmos and of all facets of our human life. Our capacities for reasoning and loving come from him, we have said. We of the Reformed tradition believe further that such a knowing and loving God, one who continually acts in us and in the world, commands our service to him by our active involvement in the life of that world.

Reconciliation, a leitmotif in Reformed thought from its earliest days to the present,[8] refers specifically to this ongoing interaction of God with his world. As Paul wrote:

When anyone is united to Christ, there is a new world; the old order has gone, and a new order has already begun. From first to last this has been the work of God. He has reconciled us men to himself through Christ, and he has enlisted us in this service of reconciliation. What I mean is, that God was in Christ reconciling the world to himself, no longer holding men's misdeeds against them, and that he has entrusted us with the message of reconciliation. We come therefore as Christ's ambassadors. It is as if God were appealing to you through us. In Christ's name we implore you, be reconciled to God. (2 Cor. 5:17–20)

God is continually renewing nature, humanity, and history: he seeks to restore alienated persons to the ground of their being. He integrates the broken psyche. He heals broken relationships between persons. He urges us to restore a respectful interaction with nature.

For Barth, Jesus Christ was reconciler and mediator. He is the Grace of God. He is the Being of Man. He has broken down the dividing wall of hostility and created the new man (Eph. 2:14). God has crossed the abyss to us in our misery, sickness, sin, and death. Christ has taken on our life in all its resistance and disorder and given it back to God new, fresh, and whole.

The healing power of the spirit of God is antagonized when we resist its blessing and impede its movements. The Hippocratic physicians were trained to "lay hands" on the sick. This action has a twofold significance: first, it conveys the trust that "you are in my hands" and that no destructive power would "lay hands on you"; second, it mediates the divine therapy. We can wish to be well and yield receptively to the healing balm of God's spirit. We can also shout "hands off" and determine to make it on our own.

In both healing and caring we see the ambivalence of human action. We know that these powers (*sōtēria* and *agapē, salus* and *caritas*) come from God. There is no other source for these energies. We can mediate them if we acknowledge the source and disavow our own power. We can also block the release of life and love into our own life and the lives of those we contact.

The presentation of this reconciling message is a healing, restoring act. We announce that the old hostility is gone, that the separating wrongs have been put right and forgiven, that friendship has been reestablished. More profoundly, it is a call from God's depth to our deep need (Ps. 42:7, 130:1). It is a message from home, that base of our life where we belong, from which we have come, where we are safe and well. The ambassador is one who is in firsthand touch with the home base, with its information and its resource. He conveys message and substance from that place. It is not a distant promise or an elusive hope that he brings. Christ himself is his own word and work. He wills to do it in partnership with us, but all our actions are instrumental to his own self-presentation.

At the end of Matthew's Gospel, Jesus tells his disciples: "Full authority in heaven and on earth has been committed to me . . . go forth therefore . . . . assured, I am with you always, to the end of time" (Matt. 28:18 ff.). The power to rescue and to heal is located in Christ and entrusted to us in this great commission. We go not in our own power but in his uncanny but certain presence, with us till the end of time.

The reconciling character of God undergirds, indeed mandates, the healing and caring mission of humanity. This doctrine of God guards the activity of healing from the dangers both of magic and shallow manipulation and of the type of caring that arises from sentimental paternalism and mechanical routine.

Persons who have been called to new being in Christ are made ambassadors. We now serve as ministers in the service of God's prophecy (*minister-ium verbi divini*). We are messengers and embodiments of the word of reconciliation. This role as instruments of the divine therapy involves word and touch, spiritual and physical care.[9] Though the designation must be used with supreme care, it is clear that we are called to cooperative, synergistic work with God in Christ. The work is reconciliation. We are invited to ambassadorial tasks. We do not go out in our own authority or with self-conceived purpose. We bear a portfolio that enables us to introduce the one whom we represent and to proclaim and live out his message.

REDEMPTION

The ultimate purpose of God's reconciliation is redemption, a bringing of all things to consummate reunion. The Hebrews borrowed the word "redemption" from secular coinage. *Goel*, redeemer or avenger, meant the purchase back of something originally owned, as when a son who sold himself into slavery to pay a debt is repurchased by the father. A ransom (*kopher*) is paid to bring back one who was lost. Deuteronomy, Psalms, and Second Isaiah used the word to describe God's delivery of his people from Egypt (Exod. 6:6, 15:13; Deut. 7:8; Ps. 106:10) or his reclamation of his people from Babylonian exile (Isa. 44:22–23). Job knew that his avenger (*goel*) lived and would vindicate his life at the last.

> I know that my Redeemer lives, and at last he will stand upon the earth;
> After my skin has been thus destroyed, then from my flesh I shall see God.
> (Job 19:25–26, my translation)

Jesus understood his life as redemptive act when he applied the sacrificial servant song in Isaiah to his own career (Mark 10:45; Isa. 53: 5–6, 10). Peter's First Epistle claims that Christ's blood in death is the ransom (*lytron*) of humanity. Paul uses the noun "redemption" (*apolytrōsis*) for the atoning, delivering work of God (Rom. 3:24, 8:23; 1 Cor. 1:30; Eph. 1:14).

In the profound experiences of suffering and dying, humans come to grips with the ultimate meaning of their own lives. The nature of God as redeemer imbues suffering with redemptive possibility and makes it into a crisis demanding interpretation and response. God as redeemer allows us to see the great value of life, for we were bought at great price (1 Cor. 6:20), thereby leading us to cherish each moment of existence. He also discloses to us that life's ultimate meaning does not lie on this side of our death, allowing us to evaluate death in its mystery and meaning. As in the natural world preservationist and entropic principles operate whereby nothing is lost in creation as end time approaches from the future, so we trust that all will be brought to its final purpose as God's will indeed consummates this reality.

Karl Barth never finished the projected fifth volume of *Dogmatics*, on "Redemption." The fragments we have from the latter parts of the fourth volume concern ethics and the doctrine of reconciliation. The heart of this material was to have been an analysis of the Lord's Prayer as our call to God from which we arise to watchful service in the world. The exposition of those great petitions "thy kingdom come, thy will be done" and "lead us not into temptation" (Matt. 6:9–13) might have informed the final section on redemption. The leitmotif of this final section was to have been faithfulness: God's faithfulness to us and to his world; our faithfulness to the community. The doctrine of reconciliation was evidently undergoing an eschatological transformation in Barth's mind as he approached death. The history of this world, of the human family, of the church, was, like his own life story, ultimately comprehended only in the final culminating intentions of God. In the suffering of disease, which vitiates both the resistant and the responsive will, and in death, which silences both our cry against and our call upon God, we are drawn into the ultimate mystery of his consummating will. As we stand mute before God, Jesus Christ, our vindicator, stands alongside as both our call and God's answer.

That we are not extinguished, that nothing is lost in the story that God has begun, is the reason we can look for meaning in suffering and for new life in death. Although the demand for redemptive significance in suffering and the belief in the necessity of immortality belong more to the logic of rational philosophers than to biblical theology, John Hick rightly claims that

... a God of infinite love would not create finite persons and then drop
them out of existence when the potentialities of their nature, including
their awareness of himself, have only just begun to be realized.[10]

The Calvinist tradition that has given most detailed attention to the doctrine of God as redeemer is the Dutch Reformed. The covenant of redemption *(pactum salutis)* (Zech. 6:13) was the arrangement between God,
Christ, and his elect parallel to, but serving a more particular purpose
than, the general covenant of grace. God in his economy initiates, Christ
executes, and the Spirit applies this salutary undertaking. Christ is the
assurance of this redemption *(engyos*: Heb. 7:22–25). He is able to save ab-
solutely those who approach God through him; he is always living to plead
on their behalf (v. 25). In Christ, sin unto death is not just overlooked, as
with the Roman *fidejussor* (forgiveness now, payment later). Christ is ex-
promissor. He has overcome sin and death in his righteous life and sacrificial death. "Death ... thou shalt die," wrote John Donne. While, for the
time being, death's terror and its premonition in suffering hold sway over
our life, our real life in Christ has already seen the force of death vanquished:

... sin pays a wage, and the wage is death, but God gives freely, and his
gift is eternal life, in union with Christ Jesus our Lord. (Rom. 6:23)

Berkhof has summarized the two main features of the Dutch Calvinist
doctrine of redemption: first, Christ has assumed our human nature, its
weaknesses and infirmities (Heb. 2:10–15; Gal. 4:4, 5; 2 Cor. 1:5–7)—
through his suffering he has achieved our redemption; second, God has received his work, delivered him from the power of death and given him eternal lordship over his company (Isa. 42:1–7; Ps. 16:8–11; Acts 2:25–28).[11]
The concept of God as redeemer has undergone numerous mutations in
modern theology. In recent empirical and process thought, God has been
removed from the older tradition, where he was aloof and apathetic from
human sufferings to a participation in human pathos and struggle.[12] While
this new direction very helpfully corrects the nonbiblical concept of Hellenistic metaphysics and Protestant orthodoxy wherein God was distant,
impersonal, and unaffected by human crisis, it really has not added to tra-
ditional theology because the passionate, pathetic God was always present,
especially in the earliest theology. Indeed, the weakness of process thought
is that God is often rendered impotent against suffering and death. While
human freedom and sin have rendered suffering and death hard and ex-

cruciating, they are exactly that (*excruciare*). They are taken out of us and up onto Christ's cross. They are not thereby made easy; if anything, they become more intense, since they are joined now to the deeper cosmic pathos (Rom. 8:22–25). Freedom and sin have now been transformed into the redemptive drama of God.

Humans either receive and share redemption as Christ offers it, or they try to make sense of suffering and death on a human plane, or they relegate them to absurdity. When we choose to go it alone, we often commit ourselves to creating biomedical utopias that attempt to ameliorate the resultant enigma of suffering and death. In the imagery of the Lord's Prayer, we can seek to let God's heavenly kingdom be manifest on earth or we can substitute some contrivance of our own. In the Reformed tradition, the prayer for "kingdom come" becomes active task, although tension is always maintained between the transcendent referent and the secular attainment. The Reformed theologian H. Richard Niebuhr has contrasted this line of approach, which was Augustine's, Calvin's, and Maurice's, with other strands of Christian tradition in terms of how Christ is related to secular culture. In contrast to views where Christ and culture are viewed in perpetual antagonism (Tertullian, Tolstoy), or synthetically accommodated (Gnosticism, Abelard, Ritschl), or distinguished by overriding transcendence (Clement, Aquinas), or juxtaposed in perpetual paradox (Marcion, Luther), the Calvinist tradition seeks constant transformation of culture under the impact of Christ's redeeming spirit.

> . . . [Calvin's] more humanistic views of the splendor of human nature still evident in the ruins of the fall, his concern for the doctrine of the resurrection of flesh, above all his emphasis on the actuality of God's sovereignty, all these lead to the thought that what the Gospel promises and makes possible as divine (not human) possibility, is the transformation of mankind in all its nature and culture into a kingdom of God in which the laws of the kingdom have been written upon this inward part. But in this case also the eschatological hope of Christ's transformation of mankind's ruined life is turned into the eschatology of physical death. . . .[13]

Niebuhr continues by questioning, righting, Calvin's concept of the human life-world in this cosmos as an intermediate testing zone suspended between eternal heaven and eternal hell. That is, Calvin considered this life as neither completely secular nor completely spiritual. Yet it cannot be doubted that Calvin, and the tradition, have taken with utmost seriousness human responsibility in the secular arena of politics, commerce, science, and technology.

Dreams of biological and technological utopias where suffering has been ameliorated and death is assaulted if not defeated proliferated in the centuries following the Renaissance. Many of these dreams were created under religious inspiration. Puritanism and Enlightenment philosophy constructed fantastic visions of new worlds where knowledge would cover the earth as the ocean waters (Isa. 11:0). Here, health would flourish, life would be prolonged, the plagues would be stopped (Jonathan Edwards), and moral and spiritual reform would transform the earth into paradise.

Secular thinkers have envisioned the same amelioration of evil and the achievement of a better world through science and politics. We now live in an age when these dreams have turned sour. All of the nineteenth-century utopias have twentieth-century mutant forms that are better called dystopias. The divine some-place transformed into a secular no-place is now a bad-place. Most of the dystopias in modern literature are biomedical. They have to do with frightful genetic and eugenic manipulations as in Huxley's *Brave New World,* or mind manipulation as in Kesey's *One Flew Over the Cuckoo's Nest* and Burgess's *Clockwork Orange,* or suspendend animation and technological distortion of the death process as in Cooke's *Coma.*

The recurring theme of this prophetic literature is that human schemes to remake man, to ameliorate pain, to conquer death ultimately harm and destroy. The only force that can save us from these horrific scenarios is a moral and spiritual vision of what the human future in the redemptive plan of God is meant to be. The most sublime imaginings of human reason or the concoctions of our malevolence portend only destruction. We need some vision of what suffering and death mean. We need a guiding theological vision.

CONCLUSION

The tenets of belief that emerge most strongly from this brief summary of Reformed theology are few in number but powerful in impact. First, the cosmos coheres in Christ, the revealed Word, God. As all meaning is found in him, the model for our "health" (that is, our existence as human persons) is Christ. His lordship provides the paradigm of, and direction for, the fully human life. Second, God is continually acting in a healing and restorative way in human history. Third, because we are God's partners in the on-going process of the redemption of this world and this time, we are to apply our reason and our compassion to healing, changing, and sustaining that world as we understand God would intend us to do. With such a world view a person is not allowed to stagnate or withdraw, for God is urging him to use his reason, to love and to serve other persons, to question, to badger, to bewail, to explore, to embrace, and to question again. In ruling, reconciling, and redeeming his cosmos, God is working out his purpose to make all things new.

Part II

HOW SHALL WE ACT? HUMAN LIFE

In the three chapters that follow, ten aspects of human life are examined: well-being and dignity, suffering and madness, passages and sexuality, morality, healing, caring, and dying. As each of these is considered in turn, it will be seen that a person or a people steeped in the theological tradition that we have elucidated as "Reformed" does carry a set of presuppositions, a way of considering the world, to the decision-making process. In this view, the active being of God imparts value to human beings. Values, seen in terms of self-estimate (well-being) and mutual esteem (dignity), emerge from God's self-disclosure. The being of God provides the ideal against which the life of the individual is to be measured: the person strives to realize the potential for loving and maturing that lies within his God-given soul.

The Reformed perspective, then, whatever its individual variations within the life of the church, is a theological perspective, one which sees the universe and time as lying within God's providence. Since history belongs to God, the person is responsible not only to realize his own gifts but to involve himself in the life of the world. The ten themes we will explore cover the full range of human experience from birth to death. There is no part of human life that lives outside the interest and concern of the Christian who belongs to the Reformed tradition; he makes decisions in his own life and reaches to help others in certain ways that we will recognize as being influenced by the beliefs we have been discussing.

·2·

Being Human:
Life's Powers and Predicaments

THE POWER OF HEALTH

WELL-BEING

All discussions of disease in any of its senses—spiritual, emotional, physical, social—asume some basic or commonly held norm of human behavior, some mode of being, against which all other behavior or modes of being are to be measured. "Disease" presupposes "ease," here spoken of as "well-being" in two of its senses, health and dignity. Well-being cannot be won or demanded from some outside source, for it exists within us as God's intention for our own life. Health and dignity point to that reality which already "is" but is hidden, distorted, or not yet fully manifest in our life. What God means us to be lies within us, if we don't ruin it in ourselves or destroy it in other people. Thus well-being (health and dignity) can be termed a human "power"—a virtue, in the Greek sense—for it waits as inherent, unfolding energy until we allow its power to burst forth.

Today, most commentary on the nature of health speaks of it as a pursuit, an achievement, a reward of personal endeavor or of sociopolitical reform. Many experts assure us that optimal health, a "state of complete physical, mental and social well-being," would be achieved if only we weed out deleterious genes, improve diets, exercise, purify the environment, detoxify the work place, or effect justice in the delivery scheme.[1]

Rather than thinking of health as a quality found in relinquishment and a gift to be thankfully received, we seek it as an assertive right. We speak of the right to life, the right to be born normal, rights of one's own body, the right to health, the right to medicare, the right to die. These are powerful assertions, affirmed quite legitimately against the deprivation of these gifts by structures and powers. But they now have become the demands of an indulged generation that does not appreciate the social commitment required to remove those evils and establish the goods we call rights. These rights are now posed as needs that someone else has the obligation to fulfill. "We did not ask to be born into this world," it is said. "Now give us what we deserve."

The concept of "natural rights" evolved from classical thought into full articulation in the seventeenth and eighteenth centuries. In the American Constitution and Bill of Rights we find a powerful articulation of the freedoms that belong to persons. These documents speak of opportunities that must not be taken away, not commodities to be provided. When we move from an affirmation that persons have the rights of free speech, assembly, life, and liberty to the assertion that we deserve shelter, food, subsistence salary, pension, health care, and the like, we have taken an erroneous leap. While the provision of these blessings may be our obligation to others, they are not entitlements.

The escalation of presumed rights in the area of well-being quickly reaches absurdity. Do we have the right to have as many children as we want—with society having the obligation to provide for them? Do we have the right knowingly to give birth to defective children, claiming that society is then obliged to care for them? The right to health quickly passes into the right to a good life when the line between necessities and luxuries is blurred. Does the right to live entail the obligation to be kept alive? Does the right to die oblige assistance in euthanasia?

The underlying model here is that of the "Athenian man," perfect in mind and body, a perfect person in a perfectly run state. That this model is "utopian," a "no-where" in which enormous price would be exacted to achieve the desired results, few (after reading Aldous Huxley and studying Nazi Germany) would deny. The technological atrocities enacted in this century surely have challenged the assumption that mankind is "progressing" or "evolving" toward perfection as he acquires mastery over nature.

To embrace a "Jerusalem" rather than an "Athens" model of man (in Dietrich Ritschl's very helpful phrase) opens a fresh vista in defining what our norm of health is to be. Basically, this view allows great flexibility, for it includes at once a conviction that one should constantly work toward improving one's world—hence the commitment of many Reformed thinkers to peace movements, ecology, political reform (or at least political involvement), social justice, and the like—and a realistic awareness that perfection is not an attainable, perhaps not even a desirable, goal. The Jerusalem man, of course, is Christ, who was "despised and rejected," who spent forty days in the wilderness in anguished spiritual torment, who suffered unjustly and died a thief's death in great physical pain. Few today would recommend seeking out suffering and martyrdom, or would willingly prolong physical or mental torment, in order to conform to this image of Christ. But accepting imperfection and finitude as perhaps necessary components of "health" may turn the search away from obsession with total social change, with complete defeat of disease (or even of death), and with the social ideal of "normal," "beautiful" and (probably) "young" persons. Human life is surely meant to be more varied and rich than the image peddled by the Barbie and Ken dolls.

Health in the Reformed Tradition

Such simple statements about the Reformed concept of health (that it includes both a drive toward discovery, cure, and reform and a sensitivity to human imperfectibility) must be fleshed out, obviously. The Reformed faith has always been a faith of transformative tension, as Richard Niebuhr put it in *Christ and Culture*. We must see how this can be so.

The Reformed tradition embraces two propositions: that life is to be received and enhanced, on the one hand, and that we "take no thought" and "seek first the kingdom," on the other. The primitive ethic found in Noachian law imputed health or wellness to harmony with natural and spiritual forces, and sickness to curse or transgression of any prohibition (i.e., taboos). In Plato, virtue created health. Just as in Hopi Indian thought a sunward soul would bring forth good action, while one turned away from the sun brought forth evil, so in Plato righteousness (well-being) was found when the facets of the soul—courage, wisdom, self-control—functioned harmoniously. The disordered soul inevitably yielded bitter fruit, while the ordered life was one of health and peace (see *Republic*, 353).

The Old Testament claims that well-being, health, happiness, fertility, and longevity are divine blessings postulated on obedience and righteousness in the people. Likewise, God guards his faithful against hunger, pestilence, and disease (Exod. 15:26). The Mosaic Code has been called a prophylactic instrument sustaining cleanliness, hygiene, leisure, human reciprocity and care—indeed, all the ingredients that make for well-being.

Jesus proclaimed and acted upon his Father's purpose of wellness and salvation for all his children (John 3:16, 10:10). He brought wholeness (salvation) to people. Whether sickness was thought to be rooted in sin, blindness (Mark 8:22–61, 10:46–52), moral laxity (John 4, the Samaritan woman), chronic illness (Mark 2:3, the Capernaite paralytic; 5:25–34, the woman with hemorrhage), or demonic possession (Mark 5:2, the Gerasene demoniac), he healed all their diseases (Mark 3:10). The apostolic community and the early church placed healing in a central position.

Very early in Christian history, indeed in the apocalyptic ethos of the

Gospel writers themselves, a mood emerged that bore on the theme of well-being. A pessimism about this world and its prospects was found in the exilic writings of the Old Testament and in Hebrew literature under Roman occupation. The Evangelists, expecting an imminent end, also discounted this world, this body, and this life when viewed against the splendor of the transhistorical kingdom of God that was announced in Jesus's ministry and provided in his resurrection. This world-transcending spirit left a profound mark on world history and made an indelible imprint on a Christian theology of medicine. Jesus said: "Do not fear those who kill the body, but cannot kill the soul. Fear him rather who is able to destroy both soul and body in hell" (Matt. 10:28). In the nineteenth century F. D. Maurice restated the claim of the Christian ages, a claim that troubles medical enthusiasts and utopians: "The weal of the body must always be subordinate to the weal of the soul."[2]

For Augustine well-being was an appropriate priority in devotion. Echoing the primitive Christian notion found in the *Didache*, that there is a way of life and of death, Augustine constructed the majestic system of the two loves, the two cities. Health and life are found in membership in the *civitas dei*. Augustine's paradisiacal man is physically and spiritually well:

> Man lived in Paradise as he desired, whilst he only desired what God commanded, he enjoyed God from whence was his good: he lived without need, and had life eternal in his power, he had meat for hunger, drink for thirst, the tree of life to keep off age, he was free from all bodily corruption and sensible molestation; he feared neither disease within nor violence without: height of health was in his flesh, and fullness of peace in his soul. . . . They were neither weary of leisure, nor unwillingly sleepy. (*C.D.* 14.26)

In Augustine all of the elements of the Western social ethic of health care are laid down. The goal or ideal is established in terms of a salutary state (paradise) that has been lost. The forces of self-will and self-love that contort this primeval well-being are identified. An interim societal strategy is commended for this time being between Fall and consummation: a political approximation of that justice that was and will be in the ordered life of adherence to natural law and the establishment of the righteous empire (the Christian commonwealth). With intelligence, creativity, and justice we will do the best we can in ensuring a good life for all. But ultimately, personal health and societal well-being are not available to the *civitas terrena*. Under the conditions of finite existence and the sin-permeated polis, the best we can hope for is minimized misery and the mediated grace of life eternal through the sacramental life of the church.

While Augustine's system commends resignation in a world forever imperfect, where wheat and tares grow together, the spirit of resistance to the status quo and the desire for a renewed world is nurtured in the millenarian hope. If a pristine state of personal and communal health once was and will yet again be, surely it is our role to resist its destruction and in some part to restore or recreate its bliss. Luther and Calvin rejected the ontocratic concept of the Holy Roman Catholic Church and Empire as the procurer of salvation and the guardian of eternal happiness for people. They claimed that salvation, vivid and accessible, is available to everyone. They recapitulated the Augustinian vision of a world preserved only in grace, which, while certainly not a human task or achievement, is lifted in the Reformation-Renaissance era from the realm of ecclesial determinism and control into the free creative realm of the human spirit. Calvin, at the opening of the *Institutes*, can celebrate medicine as "the illustration of the wondrous wisdom of God which earth declares" (1.5.2).

Reflecting the Calvinist and Puritan spirit, Francis Bacon declared in the early seventeenth century that the relief of man's estate, that is, the misery ameliorable through human science and social action, was a binding obligation. In New England a century later, Jonathan Edwards was reading the new experimental and experiential work of those British Renaissance thinkers influenced by Calvinism. Isaac Newton, Robert Boyle, William Harvey, Bacon and Locke had injected a spirit of inquiry, imagination, and creative utilization of the natural world into the Western mind. Edwards, a naturalist who wrote on insects, rainbows, and atoms, claimed that the workings of nature manifested the providence of God.[3] Humans should ingeniously utilize nature in the realm of secondary causes to serve human health and well-being. His support of Cotton Mather's controversial commitment to smallpox inoculation, for example, was illustrated by his own vaccination as an example to the citizens of Princeton, whose university presidency he had recently assumed. (Regrettably, he died of the inoculation in March 1758.)

The secrets of nature were being disclosed to the human mind by a beneficent deity. The human purposes to be served (including well-being and happiness) were felt to be self-evident in the conveyance of the scientific and technical power. Boyle wrote:

> I see not why the admitting that the Author of things designed some of his Works for these or those Uses, amongst others, may not consist with the Physical Accounts of making those things.[4]

Newton concluded his *Optics* with this faith affirmation, which pleads for science in the service of human need:

> So far as we can know by natural philosophy what is the first cause, what Power he has over us, and what Benefits we receive from him, so far our Duty towards him, as well as that towards one another, will appear to us by the Natural Light.[5]

The great nineteenth-century theologian Friedrich Schleiermacher sustained the Reformed view of celebrating life within life, rather than depreciating this world in favor of the next.

> The immortality that most men imagine and their longing for it seems to me irreligious. . . . They are concerned how to carry it with them beyond this life, and their utmost endeavor is for longer sight and better limbs.[6]

The Romantic mood in theology in fact exulted in this life, in emotions, physicality, sensual acuity, and longevity. God speaks to them: Whoever loses his life for my sake, he shall keep it, and whoever keeps it, the same shall lose it. Better, says Schleiermacher, to find well-being by reveling in what you have here and now. This is the intimation of eternity. His *Weihnachtsfest* delightfully portrays the sights, sounds, and smells of Christmas Eve, which are themselves spirit gifts. Wholeness or well-being is the feeling of absolute dependence. At all moments this life must celebrate the grace whereby it touches the infinite.

During the Enlightenment the human project gradually became dissociated from divine providence. Laplace found no need for the hypothesis of God to explain nature's laws of physics. Even the Puritan grace of acknowledging the Creator through his handiwork was unnecessary to a naturalist like Darwin. A spirit of optimism emerged that saw the establishment of peace, health, and happiness as a realizable human project, as the human enterprise moved "onward and upward." Reason, science, and technical art, along with the repudiation of inhibiting social structures like the church and the feudal order, would make it possible. Rousseau's *Discours sur l'inégalité* remembered a time when kindness reigned on earth, when natural fruits and herbs brought nutrition and healing, when love and contentment were common experiences. The Romantics not only recalled this paradise, they set out to recover it. The human project became the quest for health and happiness.

During the eighteenth and nineteenth centuries, common Christian people remained ambivalent toward this prospect of achieving a paradise here and now. If we read the sermons and diaries of that period, we do indeed see a hope reflected in dreams, in enamorment with new machines and the thrill of progress. At the same time children still died from infections, women in childbirth. The enduring message of the church that here on earth we have no lasting home constituted the common belief.

The paradoxical posture of resignation to the vicissitudes of this world and this life in favor of the eternal life provided in God's grace—except when those evils fell within the reach of human intelligence and control—remained the thrust of Calvinistic medical theology into the modern world. We hope for and work for well-being for ourselves, our family, our society, and our world. Yet we know all the while it will only be a fragment of that "shalom" which belongs to God alone and lies beyond this life. The Christian spirit strives first to prevent evil (disease), second to fight against the vectors of disease and disabilty, and third, to be present in care, even when our power to effect change has been exhausted.

F. D. Maurice reflected this feeling in a letter to a missionary doctor, a letter that captured this threefold approach to the quest for health and well-being. The natives of the country where the doctor worked believed that behind every disease lay a malignant power that must be appeased, that "disease and death are messengers of an evil power." "You will also perceive," said Maurice, "that there was a faith fighting in them with this, the acknowledgement of invisible protectors, powers of life." "The physician . . . as instrument of these benevolent powers, will work that instrument . . . with tenderness. Your ministry will show that God is a deliverer, not a destroyer."[7].

Freedom for life, respect for life, wrote Karl Barth, implies the will to be healthy. The will to be healthy is most present in a mood of joy and abandon. In a sense, health is found in the absence of a will to be healthy. "We must ask whether a special will for health is not a symptom of deficient health which can only magnify the deficiency by confirming it" (*Dogmatics*, III/4, p. 356). Health is the command of God, the power necessary to perform our physical and psychic functions. In wellness or sickness we are to affirm health: that wholeness of body and soul which is sustained by nature's salutary powers (sun, hygiene, exercise), human conviviality, and God's grace. We are encouraged to draw on the resources of the earth. The wholesome life-style, outlined by Lester Breslow as adequate rest, exercise, and a moderate diet, is commended. Barth reminded us that *mens sana in corpore sano* is "shortsighted and brutal" if it is not found in *societate sana*, which includes good living and working conditions. Barth concluded: "In the battle against sickness the final human word cannot be isolation but only fellowship" (*Dogmatics*, III/4, p. 363).

Schleiermacher noted that the life process characteristically alternated between *Insichbleiben* (abiding in self) and *Aussichheraustreten* (moving beyond self). A certain degree of self-abandon and receptivity makes for well-being: the Levitical and Christian wisdom of altruism evoked by self-esteem. "Loving thy neighbor as oneself" seems to be the secret of health. G. B. Shaw wrote: "Do not try to live forever, you will not succeed, spend all you have before you die, and do not outlive yourself."[8]

A psychologist, after reviewing thousands of books and articles and countless clinical reports on the epidemiology of health and disease, observed simply: "Those are healthiest who talk the most." Communication, receiving Word and words, is life, as is giving speech away. A Dominican priest riddled around the clock with terminal cancer pain found complete relief for two hours when he was asked to give a lecture on his great teacher, Saint Thomas Aquinas. At the personal level, compassion and generosity are health-giving virtues. At the societal level, benevolence, undergirded by justice, best guarantees the public health. For others, one hopes for pain-free, gift-enhancing happiness. For oneself, one hopes for the ability to craft a bearable existence out of physical and emotional suffering, whatever comes. For the world, one wants peace.

Case Study: The Search for Health and the New Genetics

On 22 July 1982, *The New York Times* published an editorial entitled "Whether to Make Perfect Humans." It would soon be possible, said the *Times*, to alter fundamentally the human species by engineering the genetic traits of the sex cells (sperm and egg).

Humanity's newfound ability to engineer genetic traits could well lead to the creation of a new species, as different from Homo sapiens as we are from the higher apes. So grave was the threat posed by such engineering that the *Times* suggested we consider "whether the human germ line should be declared inviolable." On 30 October 1982, the *International Herald Tribune* reported two biomedical breakthroughs. Scientists at the Salk Institute for Biological Studies had artificially duplicated a substance that released the growth hormone. GRF (growth hormone releasing factor), it was announced, would have an impact on "human growth and its disorders," would enable regulation of "the size and growth rate of domestic animals," might allow the manipulation of those functions influenced by that substance—"temperature regulation, appetite, thirst, sleep and wakefulness . . . even the emotions and the biology of aging."

On the same day the United States Food and Drug Administration approved the sale of insulin manufactured by genetically engineered bacteria. Since the number of diabetics has been increasing far faster than the supply of animal pancreas, this development promises greater availability of this life-saving substance.[9] We are reminded of Augustine's fanciful reflection that persons were bigger and better in primeval (pre-Deluge) times (*C.D.*15.9). The nostalgic fantasy of futuristic yearning to be no longer what we now are or to be something that we now are not will find manifold opportunities in biomedical engineering.

Finally, the human project of doing good in human genetics must not destroy humanity in the process. Man's power over nature can convulse into tyrannical power over human nature itself. To live with awe before nature, humility before fellow persons, and judgment before the divine is the only safeguard in a world where "each new power won by man is a power over man as well."[10]

The revelation of true (optimal) man in Jesus Christ will provide both merciful restraint and helpful guidance in the exercise of this scientific and technological urge. Christ is considerate, caring, humble, sacrificing, even receptive to death for others because he was God-toward. Nietzsche and the eugenicist philosophers of the Third Reich were offended by his portrayal of optimal humanity directed to pity and suffering rather than to power and survival. The mature manhood described by Paul (Eph. 4:13) is receptive (to the will of God) and reciprocal (interdependent). Paul's description might shock the Darwinist:

> As God's servants we try to recommend ourselves in all circumstances by our steadfast endurance: in hardships and dire straits; flogged, imprisoned, overworked, sleepless, starving. We recommend ourselves by the innocence of our behavior, our grasp of truth, our patience and kindliness; by gifts of the Holy Spirit, by sincere love, by declaring the truth, by the power of God. We wield the weapons of our righteousness in right hand and left. Honor and dishonor, praise and blame, are alike our lot: we are the imposters who speak the truth, the unknown men whom all men know; dying we still live on; disciplined by suffering, we are not done to death; in our sorrows we have always cause for joy; poor ourselves, we bring wealth to many; penniless, we own the world. (2 Cor. 6:4–10)

A Christian disposition toward biomedical engineering in the Reformed spirit will welcome developments that challenge the evils of sickness and debility. The development of synthesized insulin will be a great good. We will still need to work to correct the underlying deleterious genetic trait itself, but as phenotype therapy, this development is good and deserves support. It enables a person to live healthfully in spite of a harmful biological deviation. When we come to the fundamental construction of new types of human beings, however, or the overcoming of finitude and its symptoms (stress, anxiety, guilt, shame, grief, and mortal fear), we best recall the prototype human, Jesus Christ, one in whom fulfillment is a different perfection than biological and psychological indefectibility. For the time being it is best that we refrain from contriving some ideal biological *humanum*.

> We are God's children; what we shall be has not yet been disclosed, but we know that when it is disclosed we shall be like him.... (1 John 3:2)

DIGNITY

Having suggested a Reformed concept of health in terms of well-being, we find we must posit yet one more divinely grounded human norm before discussing disease in any of its forms. Certainly specific moral quandries, whether related to everyday decisions or biomedical crisis, cannot be analyzed without reference to human dignity—that is, what makes a person unique in creation: worth studying, respecting, and healing. God's creative being toward us makes us worthy. The troublesome word "soul" comes up here, and will not go away.

What is meant by "soul" is not some fairylike, ephemeral floating substance "imprisoned" by and totally discrete from the body, but rather the psyche (*psychē*), translated often as the heart of man, that is, what makes a human being human rather than merely animal. Why worry about the soul in this discussion of health? Can't physical, mental, and emotional health be discussed without such ancient baggage? No. All attempts to develop a "sanctity of life" doctrine (human dignity) on nontheistic grounds simply fail, and without a clear respect for human dignity one faces a utilitarian estimate of man: that persons are of value only according to the benefits they bring. The theological view generally, and the Reformed view specifically, is that each person receives from God the Creator life, not merely biological functioning but spiritual identity, the reflection of God himself within us, the persona, the *moi*, the self. The Scriptures speak of "the person as he or she is known to God," the "inner being" where God supplies spiritual life (Eph. 3:16). Some, wanting to avoid identifying soul with some idea such as Descarte's "ghost in the machine," would want to fix a material reality (a vitality locus) for the soul in DNA.

But soul in our interpretation, rather than needing to be located in time and space, can be adequately defined as *relational*: that is, we respect the dignity of other human persons because each possesses a unique psyche that is known and loved by God.

Theology, then, holds that the most helpful way of speaking of the soul is in terms of integrity and relationship. The soul is the quality of personality that unifies the person intrinsically and unites him with God. Some modern theologians have suggested that we reexamine the doctrine of the early Greek fathers, who held that, contrary to Gnosticism (in which "body imprisons soul"), the soul contains the body. But as Christians we look to Jesus Christ, the archetype of true humanity, to teach us about the soul and the dignity we need confer on one another.

Christ recreates God-life within us. Jesus exemplified the perfect integrity of life. His spirit acknowledged its source: Abba, Father. He affirmed its preeminence and divine originator and owner: "Do not fear those who can kill the body, but fear him who can destroy both body and soul in hell." He allowed his soul and body to be torn in crucifixion, his soul exploring the depths of hell to lead even captivity captive in himself (Ps. 68:16; Eph. 4:8). He came to give his soul, his psyche, as a ransom for many (Matt. 20:28; John 10:11). The perfect integration of truth and freedom and love in his life comments on both the nature and the function of the soul.

So man is something other than a physical, palpable, measurable body. For the ancients the uniqueness of man, as opposed to the animals, may have been suggested simply by his upright posture or his manual dexterity, but ultimately this uniqueness (this "dignity") was bound up in his ability to aspire, create, face, remember, analyze, and anticipate. Current discussions about human dignity (often focusing on problems such as the beginnings or endings of life) naturally involve discussions on the development of the brain, from brain stem to cortex, from vegetative functions to creativity and order. Building on this tendency to identify dignity with brain capacity and vitality, we have developed neurological criteria to establish when life begins and when it ends. When the fetus develops brain and nerve fibers and when neurochemical activity reaches a certain level, we have a person possessing dignity and, therefore, it is claimed, deserving protection. At the end of the life trajectory, the silent electro-encephalogram indicates the extinction of the person, and death can be declared.

This identity of soul or dignity with brain activity has its roots in Aristotle's thought as it was mediated through Thomas Aquinas. Psychologists and philosophers in the tradition of Aristotle have argued that there are successive stages in the development of the soul. Putting aside for the moment the notion of a preexistent soul or a soul that is polluted even as it is biologically formed, Aristotle and Aquinas claimed that the human (rational) soul was preceded by the sensitive and primal vegetative soul. The difficulty with this view, as with a traducian ("genetic transmission") or other views about the journey of the soul, is the relationship of the spiritual to the physical element. When Aristotle conjectured that ensoulment in the male fetus occurred at forty days as compared to almost ninety days in the female, he was reflecting empirically on certain physical movements rather than on any substantive change. Modern materialist thought has persisted in this error. Identifying the soul with movement, as Empedocles and Democritus did in ancient times, has led to defining it by its activity and thereby collapsing into the error of vitalism or mechanism. For this reason many modern thinkers (for example, David Hume, John Locke) have proposed that the soul is a function but not a substance.

The notion of Aristotle that the soul may be seen in various stages of development does correspond with the science of the brain's evolution. But, unfortunately, if we identify the soul with the brain, we are caught in the same reductionism to which the movement doctrine tended.

Abstract theories about the origin, development, and nature of the soul that omit the relational quality of psyche do not ultimately satisfy. No abstraction can comfort us when a friend or lover dies and that personality, so vividly present to us in relation (who touched us in our—what? our very soul) is gone. Vanished. What was this person? No, of course the question asked is "who" was this person. Death shakes the theories. We as humans may be accidents, incidents, in the unrolling of an essentially amoral and indifferent universe, but we feel that we are more than this.

The same misery that confounds us (the death of someone cherished) testifies to an impalpable but nonetheless perceived reality lying behind that mystery: we loved and were loved. So does the human experience tip precariously between extremes of despair and hope. We die, but we love. We relate. We relate out of our soul, our psyche. And theology suggests that this psyche, this relatedness, this love, this dignity, spring from God, the ground of our being human.

Dignity and the Soul in the Reformed Tradition

The earliest sense we have of the meaning of soul is "to blow, to cool" in Homer. Similarly, in the Old Testament the vital spirit in human life was thought to be the breath of God.[11] Beginning in sixth-century Greece, soul, psyche, was seen as the essence of human life, a spiritual quality. It was the goal of all moral endeavor to enrich the soul (Socrates). Plato divided the soul into the three spheres: vegetative, animal, and rational, with the higher soul properly called upon to rule over the subordinate parts.

The Greek word *psychē* was used to translate two Hebrew words: *ruach* ("wind") and *lev* ("heart") (e.g., Gen. 41:8; Jer. 4:19). Hebrew thinking associated the soul or life with the blood (Gen. 9:4) and the person (Gen. 2:7). But it was finally the heart, "the soul in its inner worth,"[12] that came to be viewed as the center of life and the epitome of the person. The heart as an instrument of moral action was an idea that came from Egypt. Memories and commandments were written on the tablets of the heart. King Tut's heart was represented on his death casket and in the *Book of the Dead* inscriptions as being removed and weighed in the underworld. His rising was contingent on the righteousness of that heart.

In the New Testament the soul (*psychē*) was closely related to life itself (*zoē*). The soul is gained by giving it away. Like well-being and sexuality, the soul is a gift received from God, a gift to be given back and given away. He who loses his psyche will save it (Matt. 10:39). The Bible calls on us to hate our soul (Luke 14:26). These strong words surely mean that we not seek to possess our life and thus destroy it. In allowing God to take hold of our heart and render it loyal to him and tender to the neighbor, it is saved to eternal life.

In the early church the doctrine of the immortal soul prompted deep respect for life. Abortion and child exposure were condemned because of the assault these acts made on eternal souls. When Augustine tried to differentiate a Christian philosophy of the soul from that in the work of Porphyry and the Neoplatonists, he claimed that the soul had a temporal beginning but no end (*C.D.* 10.31). Augustine was clear that once a human organism is formed (forty days), there is an ensouled being, bearing dignity and defying assault. Before that there is no soul. The soul is not preexistent; it is not carried in the germ cells.

> One cannot be said to be deprived of a soul if one has not yet received a soul.... There cannot be said to be live soul in a body that lacks sensation [yet unformed].[13]

Contraception and inducing miscarriage by abortifacient drugs in the first days of gestation may be morally wrong in an Augustinian view if these actions have been motivated by cruel will or false love; these are not judged because the soul is destroyed.

The significance of the soul for Augustine is the divine claim it implies and the interhuman respect if merits. The suffering, dying, and rising of the mediator savior has cleansed the soul for its return to God. The life of Christ as capsulizing the destiny of Israel is the "universal way of the soul's freedom" (*C.D.* 10.31). But Augustine was not impressed with Eastern (e.g., Persian and Indian) notions of the migration and transmigration of souls. Souls need bodies, he believed. We honor the lives of persons not because the pure soul will be damaged by harm to the body but because God in Christ has dignified the whole person by choosing the human form to bear the soul. Any concept of a pure, ethereal, disembodied soul is not in Augustine's vocabulary. Augustine's broad and subtle discussion on the human soul allows for no disembodied spirits. It is designed to affirm the entire human being. The priest who boasted of the ten thousand "souls" in his parish may be shortchanging the "whole counsel of God." The concept of an integrated self—body, mind, and soul—and the interactivity of all its structures and functions, is Augustine's lasting contribution to modern thought. In formulating its ideas on human dignity and hence struggling to define "soul," the Reformed tradition bypassed the mysticism, the body-mind dualism, and the notions of soul commerce held during the late Middle Ages, embracing instead Augustine, whose views were seen as nourished in biblical springs of truth.

Knowledge of God, said Calvin, is best achieved by a study of the human soul, the epitome of the divine handiwork. God's best recreation (problematic though it may be) is his making of souls. The long procession and individual progression of souls reflect their maker gloriously. The human soul, like the creation, is by nature good, Calvin believed. God made us body and soul, the earthen vessel a fit abode for the immortal spirit.

> The very knowledge of God sufficiently proves that souls, which transcend the world, are immortal, for no transient energy could penetrate to the fountain of life. (*Institutes*, 1.15 p. 184)

Although Calvin expresses an almost severe asceticism and suppression of the body in favor of the soul's serenity and salvation, the result of his theology is a worldly spirit. While the Lutheran ethos created a culture that celebrated physical life and the world, lifting worship and faith to a sublime height above life, the Calvinist ethos strained vigorously to see the soul shimmering (however dimly) through the darkness of secular life itself. It is this Calvinist insistence on sanctifying the physical, civic, and worldly dimension of existence that stimulated political doctrines such as "inalienable rights," "freedom of conscience," and "freedom of toleration." "The many preeminent gifts with which the human mind is endowed proclaim that something divine has been engraved upon it: all these are testimonies of an immortal essence" (*Institutes*, 1.15, p. 185). These beliefs are codified by law in nations where the Reformed influence was strong: England, Switzerland, Scotland, Holland, and the United States.

The generations following the Reformation took the Augustinian-Calvinistic psychology in two directions. On the one hand a rationalist tradition emerged that extolled the spiritual features of reason, conscience, and common sense. These qualities were thought to constitute the uniqueness of persons and thus were nurtured in church life, education, and politics.

The theology, morality, and piety of Protestant orthodoxy are highly systematic and rational. The divine revelation itself was construed to be "a system of doctrine" and a moral lexicon. In mental life and mental health, reason and logic were so stressed that irrationality was considered a disease. Education was considered discipline for soul edification, not merely data dissemination. The Calvinist academies in Europe and America as well as the early public schools, which were founded in the Puritan spirit, were crèches for divine tutelage in conscience and character as well as citadels for transmitting the classic heritage and the new experimental knowledge. Politics, following Calvin, was an ambivalent enterprise. Often communities became oppressive theocracies with elders enforcing moral uniformity and discipline. In other situations, the "toleration" ethos prevailed and the social order moved in a decidedly secular direction.

The Renaissance-Reformation also moved in a Romantic direction. The baroque mood in architecture, literature, and music reflected the Reformed spirit, extolling lyric wonder and adulation of the soul and its inventive expression in the arts. Johann Sebastian Bach sought to take the Renaissance forms of music to a new earthly perfection, where they would imitate the divine music of the spheres. While he felt he could never penetrate that curtain, his music, like Mozart's, was "always moving, free, and liberating because wise, strong, and sovereign. . . . He knew something about creation in its total goodness" (Barth, *Dogmatics*, III/3, p. 298). In Bach's splendid cantata "Wachet auf! Ruft uns die Stimme!" he depicted, through use of the parable of the wise and foolish virgins (Matt. 25:1–13), the marriage of Christ and the soul: "So come in with me, thou chosen bride. Forget, O Soul, the anguish and pain which you have to suffer." Such an overpowering union as that of the soul with its ultimate source, Christ, is ours when we glimpse eternity itself through the music of Bach or Mozart.

The Romantic mood both blessed and endangered Western culture. It infused the culture with rich spiritual expression as it aspired to creative endeavors. In absorbing soul into matter it also paved the way for a new dissociation of soul and life, which was then capitulated by the modern secularist tradition. Only today, thanks to the insights of modern biblical scholars and Karl Barth's *Dogmatics*, is our culture, especially scientific and medical culture, being reclaimed from this harmful separation of soul and body. If soul and body constitute one whole, as Augustine and Calvin suggested, then every person possesses a worth, a dignity, which must be respected.

When Hitler came to power, he was sweeping into a culture whose *Zeitgeist* was prepared for his diabolic intervention. While the Augustinian-Lutheran concept of two kingdoms has been blamed for splitting historical reality and thus abandoning this present world to evil, the seeds that grew into the Third Reich more properly can be found in eighteenth- and nineteenth-century Romanticism, which identified human power with a world-soul. Hegel, Fichte, Schelling, Feuerbach, and Nietzsche, for instance, spoke of unbridled will to power as "soul-full life." Barth wrote his commentary on Paul's Letter to the Romans and his book on theology in the nineteenth century on the eve of the First World War, as the full demonic power of this ideology was becoming manifest.[14] Barth's thrust was to reclaim the human soul to its home in Christ's transcending Lordship, tearing it away from any idea of a "passion" for some historic world-soul that united blood, race, and soil. Man "lives the healthy or sick life of his soul in his body and with the life of his body . . . so that their mutual relationship is . . . a matter of his own life history" (*Dogmatics*, III/4, pp. 358–59). Barth thus reaffirmed the integrity of body-soul unity wherein, graced with both judgment and identification, one would not sell his soul.

The Reformed tradition has affirmed that human dignity resides in our status as unique and valuable creatures of a creative God who has made us in his image and recreated us into the new being in Christ. The divine life thus imparted to us is both the unifying texture and integration of our being and our communicative link with God. In Corinthians the body is spoken of as the tent through the life of which a temple is being constructed that will not disintegrate with the encasement.

Though our outward humanity is in decay, yet day by day we are inwardly renewed. . . . For we know that if the earthly frame that houses us today should be demolished, we possess a building that God has provided. . . . we groan indeed, we who are enclosed within this earthly frame; we are oppressed because we do not want to have the old body stripped off. Rather our desire is to have the new body put on over it, so that our mortal part may be absorbed into life immortal. God himself has shaped us for this very end. (2 Cor. 4:16–5:10)

The soul is therefore our being present to God in the Holy Spirit. The soul is of moral quality. The soul is "what man is up to." God looks upon and understands the heart. Out of the heart flow the issues of life (Ps. 44:21; Jer. 17:10). The heart can be present to God as clean, wise, upright, and merry (Prov. 15) or impure, foolish, wicked, and morose (Prov. 6:18).

The soul, thus, is a generate phenomenon. It can grow into goodness; it can degenerate. God as recreator of life can plant a new heart where there is stone (*sklērokardia*) (Ezek. 11:19). When we die, we die body and soul. When God remakes us from the disintegration of death, he makes a completely new being (I Cor. 15:42 ff.). The distinctiveness of the soul is not found in either substance or function. Its dignity is not natural and intrinsic; it is alien. God gives the soul its dignity. It is distinct and inviolable because it belongs to him.

One implication of this understanding of the soul is that a person is irreplaceable. We could not clone a replica person—the body, the shell, perhaps, but not the self. A couple I know left their son for dead and handed him over for devastating experimental surgery. Doctors wondered why the parents consented to this experimentation. It turned out that they were expecting another child. They believed they had created a replacement for their severely handicapped son. In their desire to have a healthy child they did not realize that a person cannot be replaced, that their abandoned child was unique. A new baby may be a blessing for a family who has lost a child but that live baby does not duplicate the dead one, or erase the imprint the first personality made on his family.

Today we are fascinated with identifying and copying characteristics. We are gradually decoding and arranging gene sequences and will one day be able to replace defective genes and restore genetic health to a person. But we will never replace persons, even if we know and replicate all the constituent bits of information. The totality and mystery of another person is hidden in God and in the unfathomable coherence and synergy that he creates in our life.

Jung spoke of this phenomenon as individuation. The human soul is in the process of becoming. It shares qualities of consciousness with generations that have gone before. Its pilgrimage takes place in a dialectic between integration and disintegration. The unconscious, both personal and collective, is like the primal Fall, a bondage, but a bondage that is creative. The bondage to sin that Paul wrote of in Romans is something like Jung's description of the unconscious. But there is also the divine lure of the soul into grace and maturity. Becoming a self, or individuation, is "becoming a single, homogeneous being."[15]

Our respect for life is rooted, therefore, not so much in what man is but to whom he belongs and what he is becoming. An intriguing chapter in a recent book by Stanley Hauerwas is entitled "Must a Patient Be a Person to Be a Patient? Or, My Uncle Charlie Is Not Much of a Person but He Is Still My Uncle Charlie."[16] Paul Ramsey, who is being toyed with (much to his delight, I'm sure), would agree. Caring for a person because of his or her inestimable worth is the moral foundation of medical care.[17] Dignity involves our own self-esteem; our obligation to respect persons derives from the fact that we belong to God.

This perspective disallows the modern notion of valuing persons according to their neurological viability and power. The brain-vitality definition of life and death, though certainly helpful in making clinical assessments, cannot and should not become the basis for ethical and policy decisions in birth and death. Beginning with Descartes, we have thought of the human body as a machine animated by some nondescript, nonphysical entity called the soul. Identifying this entity with the function of vitality, we have almost come to the absurd point of calling the electrical-chemical discharge in the body's neurons the soul. This improves little on Descartes's locating vital contact in the pineal gland. This approach not only fails to meet the facts but tempts us to dangerous misuse of persons both by writing them off as nonpersons too soon and supporting vegetative life in failing bodies too long.

Since the atrocities of World War II, theologians, lawyers, scientists, and others have struggled anew with the concept of human dignity. The Nuremberg Code, which as the result of the postwar investigations and trials set down quasi-legal doctrine, hoped to safeguard the world from a repetition of the Nazi horrors. This code became the basis of the World Medical Association's code of ethics as well as of all subsequent professional codes and national laws regarding human investigations, such as the Declaration of Helsinki, which attempt to protect human beings from ruthless experimentation. An excerpt from that document conveys the earnestness of the desire to protect:

> The right of the research subject to safeguard his or her integrity must always be respected. Every precaution should be taken to respect the privacy of the subject and to minimize the impact of the study on the subject's physical and mental integrity and on the personality of the subject.

Our concern for human dignity, then, arises from the relationship of the individual soul, the psyche, with God the Creator. Such an affirmation affects our attitudes toward research and the treatment of human persons in the area of health and disease.

The reason and conscience of the physician, his soul, is invited to find commitment to the "health" of the patient and the "integrity" (wholeness, freedom, privacy) of the patient.

Information about the proposed intervention and opportunity to consent to that intervention must be given to the patient/subject, thus honoring the primacy of his soul in reason and will.

In life-and-death crises the physician is guardian of the health, the body-mind integrity, and the inviolability of the patient. The goals of "saving life," "reestablishing health," and "alleviating suffering" are the guiding premises of all medical treatment and research.

Public and professional ambition in the service of those same values is noble, and therefore experimentation is good and necessary. But service of the abstraction "society," either in terms of the broader community beyond the affected person or in terms of "future generations," must not override commitment to the individual patient's life and soul.

Human investigations must go on. The Reformed spirit urges us to search for ministrations that will make a whole, well, and happy life possible for all people. The imperatives of justice and mercy support us in that challenge to the evils of disease, debility, and premature death. Next to our faithfulness to God, who holds life and death, history, and the cosmos in his hands, there is no higher human purpose. To honor those generations past who gave us life and vital soul, to honor those who are now and will be our colleagues in life's journey, is the only appropriate honor we bring to God who makes and remakes us.

THE PREDICAMENT OF DISEASE

SUFFERING

As we move from the "ought" to the "is," from the real (health and dignity) to the actual (human suffering and madness), we realize how inadequate is any attempt to discuss, much less tackle, misery on either a global or a personal level. The time-tested aphorism that "the more we know, the more we know we don't know" certainly applies for anyone trying to get a grip on such topics as the springs of human motivation or the problem of evil. Disintegration dogs every effort to order the problems, and any tidy analysis may explode with the next phone call or today's newspaper headline. The very uniqueness that we lauded in defining human dignity means that, not only is there no end to the nasty surprises experience deals us and we deal each other, but also there is no bottom to our own personality, and thus perhaps no limit to our own identity with "the others."

In Conrad's "Heart of Darkness" Kurtz journeyed to the heart of the jungle, driven by curiosity about this world and his own implication in it. He discovered "who he was" in both the cosmic and the human sense, and that terrifying knowledge destroyed him. We, too, can be destroyed by discovering that "there is no health in us" or in our world, or we can continue attempting to hold knowledge and love (hope) in balance, as perhaps the narrator in Conrad's story manages to do. He knows; but he talks, he tells, he relates—that relation (to the unseen but felt audience) carrying this story, and his story, forward rather than backward into the closed shell of the self.

Thus the telling itself constitutes a kind of healing. The ordering of human problems into categories, however inadequate or overlapping these categories may be, testifies to a willingness to face evil and to spit in its face. The classic red flag raised by college philosophy teachers that "if God is good, why do we have evil (death, suffering)?" may be endlessly debated and never satisfactorily answered. Yet we, as human agents, can reply, "I know evil exists—I'm out on the wards all day—but, anyway, I can know, and love, and act." A Reformed view of the human predicament insists, as has been implied, that suffering exists in a free creation, but that humans are able to draw strength for surviving its horrors from God's love and from that love found in each other. The Reformed faith is also bold enough to claim that no suffering, however grotesque, is absurd. Even it is comprehended in the transcending meaning of our life's story.

Categories overlap throughout this study: disease, whether physical, mental, or spiritual, embraces the whole of human experience and thus can be said to subsume passages, sexuality, healing, caring, and (certainly) death. Morality refers to human action in a disordered world, hence it correlates with disease, too. But if we have recognized both this overlapping and the inadequacy of any analytical scheme, we can proceed without being stalled in a modern version of Bunyan's "slough of despond," without suffering a paralysis of our will to confront these problems boldly and to search actively for new springs that will refresh us in our struggle with the problem of evil.

"Why does it hurt so much?" A factual answer may relieve the patient's anxiety. The "why" persists, however, and strikes hard at any notion we have about justice and mercy. The biblical Job suffered unspeakable pain and grief, whether he was being cosmically "tested," as the tale suggests, or whether one day his goods or a new family were restored to him. No human attempt to answer the "why" (such as that pain is a punishment for transgressions of some kind) stops the hurting. "I must now seek out some meaning for this event in my life, why it happened to me now, at this time and with this person," a friend recently wrote after a catastrophic crisis nearly cost her life and shattered her family. This was—is—a "good" woman who did not "deserve" this anguish, who suffered all the more excruciatingly because she was an affectionate, sensitive, but strong-minded person.

Such examples are many, and our own losses or hurts are not lessened by knowing that we suffer in common with others of all places and all times. Victor Hugo's description in *Les Misérables* of the wounds at the Battle of Waterloo, *"De là une difformité de blessures qu'on n'a pas vues peut-être ailleurs"* ("These may have been the worst wounds anyone had ever seen"), shrinks from the grotesque to the comic for anyone out on the ward at Cook County Hospital, or for anyone reasonably knowledgeable about warfare as it existed long before technological sophistication refined our ways of inflicting pain on each other.

Suffering is, of course, no single phenomenon—people hurting people, or people being hurt by a malevolent universe. C. S. Lewis helpfully delineated some of the dimensions of this philosophical and theological "problem" (which is no abstraction for anyone with a dying friend) in his book *The Problem of Pain*.[18] Animal pain, he wrote, is rudimentary and universal. No animal could be said to deserve pain. Recent television programs in Great Britain have focused on the human exploitation of animals for food or experimentation. (The visual impact of that portrayal shattered the complacency of many who previously chattered away about "the food chain.")

Another level for Lewis is self-inflicted pain, represented paradigmatically by the Fall.

> When souls meet . . . they hurt one another . . . this accounts for four-fifths of the sufferings of men. . . . It is men, not God, who have produced rocks, whips, prisons, slavery, guns, bayonets and bombs; it is by human avarice or stupidity, not by the churlishness of nature, that we have poverty and overwork.[19]

The countless billions of dollars spent on weapons by all countries confound any mind aware of the horror of Hiroshima and the unrelieved world hunger of today, this very day.

We destroy our world and we destroy ourselves. We create our own diseases, as Victor Fuchs's study of health and disease in Utah and Nevada has shown. Among those communities that share a common mountainous environment, health differs drastically. Fuchs points to life-style: the Mormons, who "do not use tobacco or alcohol and in general lead stable, quiet lives" enjoy better health than do Nevada residents.[20] Despite the urgings of Ernst Wynder and the American Health Foundation, Americans continue to smoke and drink heavily and eat fatty foods, thus inflicting unnecessary pain on themselves.

Another level of pain is that of unexplained physical suffering. The condition of mortality itself seems to carry with it the requirement that we suffer from and succumb to some organ failure or infection, or some form of general deterioration, and thus physically suffer before we die. Cancer, which Freud called "the last disease," may appear not only because of our poisonous environment or harmful life-style but because medical advance has relieved or banished other diseases that might have attacked us. But this historical explanation still does not explain why a healthy, active mother who breast-fed her children and had no deleterious habits suffers and dies of cancer long "before her time." To say that such a woman lived a quality life short in years doesn't feed her children or fill her husband's lonely house. The "why" presses urgently here: and when we say goodbye to such a one we remember Ivan Karamazov's protest that he could not believe in a God who permitted little children to suffer. Even more poignant for our time perhaps is Camus's Dr. Rieux in *The Plague*, whose town is suddenly struck by an epidemic of the plague. How can one ever explain this misery inflicted at random on all ages, all conditions? Perhaps one could say that a child has passed on to a better world, one whose delights compensate for this suffering; but Rieux cries, "*Qui pouvait affirmer en effect que l'eternite d'une joie pouvait compenser un instant de la douleur humaine?*" ("Who would dare suggest that an eternity of joy would be able to compensate for one moment of human misery?").

So the discussion of suffering becomes, once again, no longer abstract, but personal, and the issue becomes not how to avoid or even eradicate suffering (it cannot be done), but how to face it.

Suffering in the Reformed Tradition

The Reformed tradition, like all religious traditions, has stimulated the human struggle against suffering and at the same time has sought to discover purpose in this experience through the nurturing of care and mutual support. We can best assess the tradition's response to suffering and suggest its future direction by surveying the developments of theodicy and a theology of patience in the Reformed heritage.

Primitive wisdom construed suffering as punishment, and health and prosperity as blessings of the gods or of the fates. Even the suffering associated with sickness was seen as reflecting some fault in oneself or in one's tribe. Cotton Mather, when he spoke of the diphtheria epidemic sweeping across New England in the eighteenth century as God's judgment on his people for falling away from their vibrant Puritan faith, was reiterating an ancient tradition.

In the biblical record we find insights concerning the source and significance of suffering. In the early stages of its existence, Israel, like all Semitic peoples, interpreted suffering as divine punishment for sin. While the wicked might do well for a time, all believed that the sins of wicked persons would eventually "find them out" and they would somehow be afflicted (Ps. 7:15–16). Later, other themes come into play; even the righteous suffer (Job, Psalms). Therefore, there is some universal judgment that falls like the rain or sunshine on good and evil alike. The price of natural law is suffering; for the cosmos, like the human will, has been created free. Sometimes God chastens through suffering (Deuteronomy, Isaiah). Suffering here becomes the vehicle for correcting and purifying. The word "pain" is actually derived from two roots: the Sanskrit *pu* ("purification") and the Latin *poena* ("punishment"). Finally, in the exilic literature, the theme of redemptive suffering appears (Isa. 40:2, 53, 55:5). The suffering servant of God takes the guilt of the nation onto himself and vicariously suffers.

This sets the stage for the New Testament's treatment of suffering, a perspective that accents all the above motifs and adds some new themes.

> . . . this is how God fulfilled what he had foretold in the utterances of all the prophets: that his Messiah should suffer. (Acts 3:18–19)

> . . . the sufferings we now endure bear no comparison with the splendor, as yet unrevealed, which is in store for us. (Rom. 8:18–19)

> . . . if anyone suffers as a Christian, he should feel it no disgrace, but confess that name to the honor of God. (1 Pet. 4:16)

The New Testament blends many kinds and many interpretations of suffering. Although the disciples, and the early church generally, were being persecuted and executed for the faith, this witness, this *martyrion* (hence, "martyrdom"), was to be welcomed. Although the healing episodes of the Gospels announce God's power over suffering, the interpretation remains mysterious. Speaking of a blind man, the disciples asked, "Rabbi, who sinned, this man or his parents? Why was he born blind?" Jesus answered: "It is not that this man or his parents sinned . . . he was born blind that God's power might be displayed in curing him" (John 9:1–4). The disciples are told to heal the sick and relieve suffering, but the healed are not to tell of their cure (Mark 8:26).

> . . . your heavenly Father . . . sends the rain on the honest and the dishonest. (Matt. 5:46)

> . . . he learned obedience in the school of suffering. (Heb. 5:8)

What view of suffering emerges from this complex picture? First, Jesus Christ has come to bring life in abundance. Faithfulness to him therefore requires that we confront the forces that inflict injury and suffering on people. The pain of disease, for example, is being drawn under his judgment, as his saving kingdom penetrates deeper into the reality of human life. The understanding of, and caring for, physical pain, as by drugs or surgery, is a noble human endeavor that enjoys the inspiration of God. Much suffering between people is brought on by our neglect and violence, our sin. Christ's purpose is to lift this self-destructiveness and malevolence from us and give us new relationships based on love, hope, and peace. Such distraction (from self) and delight in living purposefully is the best antidote to pain. Finally, Christ calls us to suffer with him, to share the burden of redeeming a world that is confused, lost, and determined to save itself. Whenever the Gospel of release from egocentricity and group aggrandizement is announced, conflict, retaliation, and suffering are provoked. This suffering is the call of Christ to join him in redemptive work. The final summary of Paul's moral instruction to the waiting community is *agapē* (self-sacrificing love), not *pleonexia* (taking, or making-do, oneself).[21]

"Come, Grace, and let this world pass away. . . . Maranantha" (*Didache* 8:6). This prayer was often found on the lips of the early Christians. Those who suffered for their witness, those for whom life had grown unbearable, those whose bodies and minds were wracked with illness, often used this prayer. The vivid and palpable sense of the fully redeemed life that waited on the other side of death has often tempered the response to suffering. This confidence has strengthened serenity, shortened patience, even abetted martyrdom and suicide. The yearning to pass from this turbulent sea of sufferings to the "blissful shore" has been strong in Christian piety through the ages. Elizabeth Kübler-Ross says she cannot tell us what she has seen on the other side of death because it is so beautiful we would all commit suicide. She is, of course, echoing the idea of the afterlife as it was depicted by medieval and Puritan preachers: eternal torments for the damned (including those who commit suicide) and eternal felicity for the righteous.

Again, it was Augustine who created for Reformed theology—indeed, for all Christian thought—the great system of theodicy and the Christocentric interpretation of suffering.[22] Henry Chadwick, the great early-church scholar (the only person in Great Britain, it is said, who has read all of Augustine), has just finished in Oxford a series of lectures on the bishop of Hippo. He argues that Augustine's principle teaching on evil and suffering is Platonism, chastened by the Gospel. Evils are not ultimately real but are rather the absence of good. Sufferings are like the patient undergoing surgery, the woman hurting in childbirth, the schoolboy agonizing over his lessons. Sufferings are the shadows in a fine painting or the dissonances in a piece of music. They are necessary, yes, providential nuances that enrich the grand picture. Miseries are the lot of humanity. The world is like a great grist mill that grinds wheat and scatters chaff. This world takes its toll. Only by clinging to Christ in salvation through the saving benefits of the church, Augustine believed, are we saved from total despair.

Sufferings are divine blessings in that they make the allures of this life distasteful and whet our appetite for God's kingdom: Augustine warned:

> When all goes well with you, when the world smiles on you, no one in your family has died, no drought, hail, or fruitlessness has attacked your vineyard, your wine-cask is not sour, your cattle haven't failed, you have not been shamed in any high worldly position, your friends all survive and think well of you, your dependents want nothing, your children obey, your slaves tremble before you, your wife is harmonious with you and the house is happy—then find tribulation—if in any way you can—that having found tribulation—you may call on the name of the Lord.[23]

"Who would not tremble and rather choose to die than to be an infant again," asked Augustine. "We begin it with tears, and therein presage our future miseries" (*C.D.* 21.14). Augustine experienced life as the Psalmist did:

> The hurrying years are labor and sorry, so quickly they pass and are forgotten. (Ps. 90:10)

Augustine lived through the great historical calamity of the fall of Rome to the barbarians, in A.D. 410. Not only was this an assault on, and in some sense a repudiation of, the Christian empire, but now *christiana tempora* have become indeed *mala tempora*. The rupture of the impressive culture established by Emperor Constantine promised only social and cultural chaos to accompany the personal misery of plague, disease, and loss.

The Middle Ages was a period when persons increasingly sublimated their sufferings into a yearning for eternity. Although secular songs and stories (for example, Boccaccio's *Decameron*) show us the delightful Dionysian side of medieval life, the great effort of the age was to aspire toward God and eternity. As the great cathedrals were constructed, the people were pouring out their hearts in soaring devotion to God.[24]

The age of Luther, Calvin, and the Renaissance-Reformation was one of plague, natural catastrophe, national upheaval, and profound internal anxiety. Calvin's doctrine of providence was formed against this background. Calvin's biographers have shown that he lived a life of constant physical suffering, with gout, kidney ailments, and other afflictions. He gathered this personal sorrow and broader calamity into a systematic understanding of providence, ignorance of which is the "greatest of miseries."[25] In a passage reminiscent of Augustine, Calvin wrote:

> Whatever kind of tribulation presses upon us, we must ever look to this aid: to accustom ourselves to contempt for the present life and to be aroused thereby to meditate upon the future life. For since God knows best how much we are inclined by nature to a brutish love of this world, he uses the fittest means (sufferings) to draw us back and to shake off our sluggishness, lest we cleave too tenaciously to that love." (*Institutes*, 3.9, p. 712)

Calvin's contempt for, and serenity in the face of, suffering has been perpetuated in the Puritan tradition by a suppression of response to physical pain and a "grin and bear it" composure that discourages expression, sharing, commiseration. This emotional characteristic of the Puritan personality can be traced to Calvin's understanding of physical suffering. He believed that Jesus' atonement has to do with spiritual, rather than physical, suffering. In one of his many sermons on Isaiah 53, Calvin wrote:

> The reason for the weaknesses, sorrows and ignominy of Christ is that he bore our infirmities. Matthew 8:17 quotes this passage after relating that Christ cured various diseases, though it is certain that he was appointed to cure, not men's bodies, but their souls.[26]

In his book *People in Pain*, Mark Zborowski notes in an extensive study of pain response among different ethnic-religious groups in a New York hospital that old Americans (including Anglo-Saxon Protestants and Calvinists) suffer in silence—this in contrast to Irish and Italian Catholics, European Jews, and others, who cry, moan, and express their pain more overtly.[27] Calvinist serenity, tending toward complacency in the face of suffering, has been a strong force in creating the age of pharmacologic pain amelioration in the modern world. The Protestant patient in the hospital wants to get rid of pain by whatever means. "Cut it out," "blot it out," and "tranquilize it away" express this mentality. The piles of valium consumed each year in the industrialized culture created in the Puritan ethos attest to the great distance we have come from Calvin. Rather than seizing on these experiences to make amends in life and draw near to God, we seek to obliterate pain and get back to our business as usual. As a result, we experience more constant and unrelenting suffering and find ourselves under almost constant sedation.

> The Lord Jesus . . . endured most grievous torments in his soul and most painful sufferings in his body; was crucified and died; was buried, and remained under the power of death. . . . On the third day he arose from the dead, with the same body in which he suffered . . . and purchased not only reconciliation but an everlasting inheritance in the Kingdom of Heaven. (Westminster Confession, 8.4.5, p. 204)

The basic thrust of the Reformed theology of suffering is that Christ has taken to himself our sin, suffering, and death, which are causally linked together in our rebellion against, and our estrangement from, God. These Christ has fully borne and endured on his own body, which deserved no suffering or death. In his victory we are released, not from the experiences of sin, suffering, and death, but from their power over us. They are taken on by the "eternally crucified one" and made forever impotent. We are thus freed to live for him in his project of reconciling the world unto himself and reconciling his inheritance, God's shattered creation. The meaning of suffering and redemption is therefore, as Barth suggested, reconciling ethics.

Gandhi and the Eastern mystics have shown us that suffering, purification of soul, and moral commitment are inextricably related. God chastens those whom he loves (Heb. 12:6). The fruitful tree is pruned in order to bear more fruit (John 15:2). The telos of suffering is discipline and deeper ethical commitment. "Plagues and pestilences," wrote Maurice, "lead to moral effort, to physical purification. Terrible wars punish money-worship and extinguish slavery. . . . Satan shall be bruised under Christ's feet."[28]

Barth added a short note about the Sermon on the Mount in his volume on reconciliation. This chapter on Christian moral existence imputed beatitude to "the poor in spirit," "those who mourn," "the meek," "the reviled and persecuted," "those who weep." After forcefully declaring how un-Hebraic it would be to label these conditions in and of themselves "blessed," Barth went on to say: "in their suffering they are seen in confrontation with the Kingdom of God" (*Dogmatics*, IV/2, p. 190). In their misery they find themselves "at the outer edge of the cosmos." Luke's malediction on the well and wealthy in his version of the Beatitudes (Luke 6:24 ff.) signals that in the healing of the sick and the saving of the suffering, as well as in the impoverishing of the rich and the striking down of the well, God is manifesting his kingdom.

"Suffering," wrote H. Richard Niebuhr, "is the exhibition of the presence in our existence of that which is not under our control . . . in response to suffering [people] define themselves, take on character, develop their ethos."[29] Part of the morally redemptive response to suffering is to draw within our responsible control those forces "out of our control" that compound the nature and inevitable burden of conditions of subservience and slavery, of intimidation and torture, racial and social deprivation: all of these impose suffering, which suffering Christians must seek to remove. James Gustafson adds other areas of "fatedness," including inherited diseases as forces from which we should properly seek redemption. "Where human agency can rectify the effects of fatedness, can bring some good out of natural evils, can create possibilities in society and culture for those who are in despair, and can alter institutional arrangements to restrain threats to human well-being and create opportunities for human flourishing, a form of redemption is occurring."[30]

Perhaps the most lively arena of redemption in our world today is that realm of newfound freedom and happiness that is developing under the impact of education, science, technology, and medicine. In the few short decades since the dawn of the age of antibiotics and immunization, countless millions of persons have been spared suffering and early death. While this has in part created the population-growth crisis (which imposes another form of suffering), this great blessing is but the first ray of sun on the horizon. We have yet to assimilate this, the "most dramatic and abrupt health change ever experienced by mankind.[31] On the horizon now is appearing another glimmer that may prove an even greater force in human redemption from suffering. The ability to understand and do something about the genetic conditions that contribute to disease will perhaps be the finest achievement of our time. Yet suffering may not be completely ameliorated. In fact, release from more basic levels of pain may make possible the experience of deeper forms of suffering. Already we are beginning to see a new epidemic of senility and other chronic diseases of the elderly.

Whether geriatric medicine and psychiatry will significantly respond to the increasing power of this vector of disease remains to be seen.

In the meanwhile, what do we hope for? In response to redeeming love, what do we set out to achieve? The theology and ethic we have studied prompts us to work energetically for the new world while waiting patiently for it. We must cease our violent coercion of nature to serve our "needs"; instead, we must gently foster its own natural and provident directions. With our biological powers we should not construct some blissful pain-free sedated humanity but use our powers to safeguard and fulfill humanity's intrinsic potential. We should not violently seek to topple the existing political structures and put in their place some new tyranny, but to transform the orders from within, with the imperatives of justice and freedom. Suffering is God's reminder to us of what is yet to be: we find in it the distance between what is and what will be. It is the "goal of the future that stabs inexorably into every unfulfilled present."[32] In the great testament of cosmic redemption, Paul writes:

> The created universe waits with eager expectation.... It was made the victim of suffering not by its own choice—but by the will of Him who subjected it in hope.... We do hope because the universe itself is to be freed from the shackles of mortality and enter upon the liberty and splendor of the Children of God." (Rom. 8:21–24, my translation)

Case Study: Suffering and Truthfulness

The resident asked me to come quickly and see the patient. The young cancer victim was very distraught. He had noticed his hospital chart on the bed with a large DNR (do not resuscitate) order written in. When I got to his bedside, he asked what this meant. I told him that this was a directive that no resuscitative measures be taken should he go into a cardiac arrest. He asked why the note had been written without consulting him. We called the whole party—doctors, nurses, family—and discussed the case with the patient. He was pleased to use this opportunity to teach us all a good lesson. The staff had not told him about the directive in order to "spare him unnecessary suffering" and "not to weaken his hope." To everyone's surprise the young man said that he completely agreed with the decision and only wished that he could have been part of it. He knew he had only a short time to live and did not want to be kept alive. If a merciful infection or even a more merciful arrest were to come along, he would like to allow these forces to carry him away. He was ready to die, both by weariness of his sufferings and by faith in God that greater life awaited him.

The Christian's calling is, first, not to cause suffering; second, to alleviate it when and where that is fitting; third, to allow suffering to do its work when it is redemptive or when alleviation will only amplify its severity and duration; and, last, to stand closely by those who suffer, pleading their plight to God and to those who might help, and in the end being with them in sympathy and empathy. In his mass on the world, Pierre Teilhard de Chardin prayed:

> This restless multitude, confused or orderly, the immensity of which terrifies us; this ocean of humanity whose slow, monotonous wave-flows trouble the hearts even of those whose faith is most firm: it is to this deep that I desire all the fibers of my being should respond. All the things in the world which this day will bring increase; all those that will diminish; all those that will die: all of them Lord, I try to gather in my arms, so as to hold them out to you in offering.[33]

MADNESS

Madness represents the dark underside of human dignity. Some initial distinctions must be made here: first, that while mental and/or spiritual pain may be as excruciating for the sufferer as physical pain, they are of different orders; second, that physical pain is easier to measure, analyze, and relieve than are mental and spiritual pain. Further, mental or spiritual torment are sometimes thought to have positive "benefits" (for the individual or for society) that are rarely attributed to physical pain.

The edges of "normaloy" fray in tailoring any definition of madness. As Shakespeare recognized, one who functions perfectly well in ordered society may be the "madman" according to some "higher" definition of sanity, as Lear is "mad" not only when he raves on the heath,

> . . . he was met even now
> As mad as the vex'd sea; singing aloud;
> Crowned with rank furmiter and furrow-weeds. . . .
> (*King Lear*, IV, iv, 1–3)

but when he reigns in the summit of his power, a stranger to compassion. Kent strikes home, identifying Lear as both "mad" and evil-doing, that is, "diseased" in casting off his daughter Cordelia (I, i, 147–69). Here, the "higher" definition of sanity is the realist's insistence that life and relationship continue despite death and that love is the greatest human "treasure."

Who is the "madman" in the inverted world of *Twelfth Night*? Is it the cynical fool, the cloistered Olivia, the love-struck Duke, the empty-headed

Sir Andrew, or the imprisoned Malvolio? Shakespeare plays with varying interpretations of mental and spiritual disintegration as he questions how to measure the normalcy against which madness is to be defined. The scene in which Malvolio is chained in a darkened room in an effort to make him doubt his own senses exposes the fragility of all our definitions. The audience has already been told that Malvolio is being "fooled"—that is, he is not "clinically" insane, despite all efforts to drive him to desperation. But spiritually (again, operating according to the playwright's underlying vision of affection, fun, and joy as "sanity") Malvolio must be judged diseased, insane. Sir Toby exclaims, "Dost thou think, because thou art virtuous, there shall be no more cakes and ale?" (II, iii) and Malvolio's parting cry for "revenge" marks his spiritual alienation from any affirming elements that might aid the ongoing human story.

Shakespeare, like Goethe, Calvin, or Saint Paul, recognized the inherent doubleness of the human *psyche*, the mind or "soul" (in Bruno Bettelheim's translation of Freud's concept of psyche). Man's will, wrote Calvin (building on a pseudo-Augustine text) is like a horse carrying one of two riders: God or the devil. The one rides gently, safely, on the right course, the other "violently drives it far from the trail, forces it into ditches, tumbles it over cliffs, and goads it into obstinacy and fierceness" (*Institutes*, 2.4, p. 309). Only the good rider can lead it safely. The diseased mind or soul tears in opposite directions; the healthy or "sane" one symbolically unites in pulling in one direction. In Socrates's language, the soul is only safe when possessed by a good demon; diabolic life yanks the self away from integrity and coherence into the ditches of disintegration and chaos. Jesus said, "Take my yoke upon you, my burden is light. You shall find relief for your soul" (Matt. 11:29–30).

To treat briefly in Reformed perspective the theme of madness or the life of the mind we will take Paul's searching description of the tortured existence of the human psyche in Romans (7:14–8:2), and in the light of Reformed exegesis in Augustine, Calvin, and Barth, we will relate this understanding to the unfolding knowledge of sanity and madness as it is developing in modern medicine and psychiatry. In particular, we will consider the work of two psychiatrists who, in differing degrees, have come under the influence of the Calvinist tradition: the Scot Ronald Laing and the American Karl Menninger. Finally, our case study will focus this theological and medical insight on the moral dimensions of mental illness.

Paul's description of the plight of the psyche as detailed in Romans 7 serves as a normative background for understanding and evaluating both mental health and madness in a Christian perspective. Only such a normative standard can safeguard us from therapeutic nihilism (Laing, Szass), which on the basis of optimism about man sees mental illness as myth, and from behavioral management therapies, which see the human mind as infinitely malleable and programmable.

The knowledge of God as recreator has made it clear that we need to be remade. That our original creation was good and that something has gone wrong is evident in our experience. Paul speaks through the experience of every person when he cries out: "I do not know what I am doing, I do not do what I want, but I do what I hate" (Rom. 7:14–15). Our experience, like our awareness of God, points out that we have become something we do not wish to be and were not meant to be. This crisis is in reason and in conscience. "I do not know . . . I do not do." The will drives on, unresponsive to both intellect and moral sense.

This passage from Romans is pivotal to Christian theology. For Augustine, Luther, Calvin, Wesley, Barth, and many other seminal Christian thinkers, it was a key to the whole system.

> There was a time when, in the absence of law, I was fully alive; but when the commandment came, sin sprang to life and I died. . . . We know that the law is spiritual; but I am not: I am unspiritual, the purchased slave of sin. I do not even acknowledge my own actions as mine, for what I do is not what I want to do, but what I detest. But if what I do is against my will, it means that I agree with the law and hold it to be admirable. But as things are, it is no longer I who perform the action, but sin that lodges in me. . . . the good which I want to do, I fail to do; but what I do is the wrong which is against my will; and if what I do is against my will, clearly it is no longer I who am the agent, but sin that has its lodging in me. . . . Miserable creature that I am, who is there to rescue me out of this body doomed to death? God alone, through Jesus Christ our Lord! thanks be to God! . . . the conclusion of the matter is this: there is no condemnation for those who are united with Christ Jesus, because in Christ Jesus the life-giving law of the spirit has set you free from the law of sin and death. (Rom. 7:9 ff.)

A debate rages today over the nature of mental illness. The newfound sciences and practices—medical psychiatry, psychoanalysis, and clinical psychology—have struggled with the question as to whether the crises and pathology of the human psyche are mental illness or moral failure. Experts have lined up on both sides of the question. Some have argued that medical psychiatry and psychology should restrict themselves to organic syndromes that have clear genetic, neurological, and biochemical derivation and respond to chemical, surgical, and electrical therapy. Those in the psychoanalytic tradition contend that the Freudian interpretation of personality (the scheme of id, ego, superego, unconscious, and psychosexual development) clarifies problems and helps us move toward constructive solutions. Others feel that the life-style, behavioral, and moral problems that people face are clinically classifiable and amenable to the therapies at hand: medication, counseling, behavior modification, and the like.

Saint Paul observed conflict and crisis at the center of both his own being and the being of every person. It is the crisis of reason, will, and conscience. It is the crisis of coming to terms with who one is and of understanding the forces at work within us. It has manifested itself in physical symptoms that have been variously described as frontal-lobe epilepsy, sadomasochism, or infantile fixation. In one sense it is a schizophrenic struggle, the war between two selves. It is also the conflict between two drives: one into life, the other toward death. The one drives deeper into self, into apathy, passivity, and disinterest, into a dissociation that verges on autism. The other opens one more to contact, adventure, and sympathy. Paul concluded that his actual self, the personality that he shared with everyone else, the natural self, was not his authentic self. The real self came to life only as the animating spirit of God introduced new life and new being into his personality. This old self reappeared even after grace had generated new existence; yet now it no longer controlled and condemned.

Augustine pondered deeply this passage from Paul. He used its insight repeatedly as he sketched the Christian doctrine of self between the errors of Manichaeanism and Pelagianism. In a word, the Manichaeans argued that human thought and action was deterministically driven, that basic causal force in nature controlled and guided all activity. The Pelagians (who, like the Manichaeans, were probably quite unlike the caricatures theologians have painted) emphasized the essential goodness and free possibility of the human spirit.[34]

Augustine, with Paul, saw man as an exile from himself. Torn between self-love and right affection toward self, God, the world, and everyone else, perpetual misery was each person's plight. The moral law, vivid within conscience and reason, continually recalled to him this discrepancy. So did the fear of death. The ubiquitous presence of law and finitude in one's experience continually goaded one into greater and greater discontent. For Augustine, the more one gets to know oneself, the less one likes what one sees. This led him to postulate the doctrine of original sin. We find ourselves at this moment continuing to sin, Augustine wrote, unable to stop. This empirical observation, related causally to all the misery in the world, constituted Augustine's concept of *peccatum originale*.

It is not from the liberty of the human will, nor from the precepts of the law, that there comes deliverance from this body of death; for both of these he [Paul] had already—the one in his nature, the other in his learning; all he [lacked] was the help of the grace of God, through Jesus Christ our Lord.[35]

Neither moral adherence nor free will, but only the grace of Christ, could save this self.

Luther and Calvin began their theological discussions of the plight of the human soul with the Letter to the Romans. Luther, after commencing his career as Bible teacher at Wittenberg with lectures on the Psalms, turned to Romans. The book was instrumental in his own soul search. In his first lectures on the Psalms he noted the dramatic insight that Romans 1:17 had given him. The phrase "the just shall live by faith" had "opened the door of paradise to him." This was the same passage repeated in his later account of the great release in the tower when he buried the devil in "dirt" by defecating on him and found his own *Seelengrund* in God's justice.[36] Luther's favorite passage in the Bible was Romans 7. Here was the clear description of man as both saint and sinner. Here was the classic text that showed the cleavage in the human mind and conscience. If Saint Paul, the noblest soul that God ever raised, experienced this inner contradiction, surely all others, myself included, will experience it as well. We, too, can overcome it in the grace of Christ.[37]

Calvin, by contrast, treated Romans 7:14 ff. serenely: Paul, he wrote, was simply stating the contrast between fleshly and spiritual motivation. God is reforming us into his own spiritual image and we resist by living according to the flesh. The whole inclination of our mind is wayward; the natural life is completely "borne away by lust." Even the godly person, for whom God is the whole desire of his heart, is drawn by the heaviness of flesh. "Flesh" here means not only sexual misdirection but the total weight of ignorance, error, misperception, and inclination and behavior harmful to self and others.[38] Here again we have the great Pauline doctrine of "ego" and "not I": "I no longer live, but Christ lives in me" (Gal. 2:20).

Paul, as Everyman, "comes from the realm of Spirit," wrote Barth, "and passes relentlessly to death."[39] Impressed in consciousness by spirit and impending death, man "is engaged inevitably and hopefully in a conflict from which there is no escape, because it is the battle for his very existence."

I see that the law which proceeds from the Spirit, compelling, necessary, and inevitable though it be, is excluded from my existence as a man. What form of human existence is competent to receive this impress, to arrange

itself according to this misery and hope, and to accept this demand? Surely
no human existence of which I have experience. What answer can I give?
How can I obey a call which has emerged from beyond the boundary of
my existence? ... Only a New man, only a victory over my humanity,
only eternal life, can release me from the enigma of my being.[40]

"If God be God, who then am I? The EGO which practices what I—the
other EGO—contemplate with evident horror, cannot be an EGO capable
of surviving the question." Like Augustine and Calvin, Barth finally decided
that this actual self was insufficient unto itself. Only when it was drawn into
the alter-self, Christ's new and restored ego, was the self restored to itself.

Much mental discomfort and disease is formed within the felt discrepancy
between the actual self and some ideal self. Anxiety neurosis, our most
common mental disorder, with its companion symptoms of depression,
tension, and agitation, quite often manifests some Pauline struggle wherein a former order is passing away and one is getting old and losing earlier
vitalities (hopes, tasks, associations), or where some unrealized ideal construct reminds us of what could and should have been. Flight to some ideal
self is madness, finding one's real self is health and peace.

In former ages madness was called melancholia, the brooding, depress-
ing, black moodiness that led persons to retreat completely from the joys
and stimulations of living. Robert Burton's 1621 treatise *The Anatomy of
Melancholy* characterized it as habitual or episodic. All of us experience
the "transitory melancholy" that is provoked by sorrow, sickness, trouble,
fear. There is also the more chronic disposition that is "dull," "sad," and
"sour." Melancholy in this sense is the "character of mortality."[41]

In addition to death neurosis, melancholy is also unsatisfied desire, unrealized ambition, and unfulfilled possibility. As such it leads to frustration
and exhaustion. But this great emotion, like the law in Paul's description,
can be both a friend and a messenger. It can take one to the limits of land-
locked existence and lead one to venture into uncharted seas. In Tolstoy's
The Death of Ivan Illich, the hero experiences profound melancholy. This
brooding pessimism leads him to dissociate himself from all the possessions, obsessions, and attractions of his former life and find spiritual meaning in "the kingdom within." It is the child's hand reaching to him on the
deathbed that finally breaks through his ego-hold consciousness and brings
ego-release and wholeness (salvation).

Madness may be defined as clinging to a driving force that is misguided
and out of control. When Socrates and Jesus spoke of madness as demonic
possession, they were recording the empirical observation that such persons
were being torn apart (cf. Mark 5:12 ff.) by conflicting, multidirectional

energies. Jesus cast out demons, drew in their diabolical reins, and gave symbolic (integral) life and health to such persons.

In the 1901 Gifford Lectures William James issued a thoughtful challenge to the view of mental health and madness we are exploring. Sick souls, he wrote, "must be twice-born in order to be happy . . . the healthy minded need to be born only once." In the lecture entitled "The Divided Self," he continued: "The psychological basis of the twice-born character seems to be a certain discordancy or heterogeneity in the native temperment of the subject, an incompletely unified moral and intellectual constitution." The world view of the "healthy minded" person is a "rectilinear, one-storied affair"; for the "sick souls" the world is a "double-storied mystery."[42] Here we have the crux of the dialogue between psychiatry and theology. Is there some sense in which the bipolar, schizoid, "divided self" personality is part of a normal moral struggle as opposed to being a pathological state?

After eighty years of tragic experience in this twentieth century of destruction one wonders whether James would see the secularized single-mindedness that verges on monomania as health. Certainly religious conversionism and salvationism have both stimulated and been stimulated by the unhealthy personality. But perhaps reality is two-storied. Perhaps there is a God who transcends, yet comes to, this earth. Perhaps on that night of nights God did descend down the back staircase of the world into the stable of Bethlehem.[43] Perhaps time and eternity, nature and supernature, are two realms that impinge on the human soul. Perhaps one who participates in these two worlds is indeed the whole and happy individual. Are soul-crisis and salvation a wholesome or a deleterious development in the person? The Gospel claims that Christ came to bring integrated, whole, unified life. This is the meaning of salvation, *sōtēria*, which connotes mending, healing (Mark 1:19).

Ronald Laing took James's title "The Divided Self" for his 1959 book. As a psychiatrist Laing was impressed with the duality of human existence. The escape from self was nothing more that Paul's flight from freedom to law.

> When the great Tao is lost, spring forth benevolence and righteousness. When wisdom and sagacity arise, there are great hypocrites. When family relations are no longer harmonious, we have filial children and devoted parents. When a nation is in confusion and disorder, patriots are recognized.

This escape from freedom into moralism is nothing less than the division of the self:

> Once the fissure into self and ego, inner and outer, good and bad, occur, all else is an infernal dance of false dualities. It has always been recognized that if you split down the middle, if you insist on grabbing this without that, if you cling to the good without the bad, denying the one for the other, what happens is that the dissociated evil impulse, now evil in a double sense, returns to permeate the good and turn it into itself.[44]

From this dualistic assumption, Laing proceeded to argue that many of our designations of persons as mentally ill, and our inhuman institutionalization and mistreatment of the insane, are merely political control and moral containment. We are "all murderers and prostitutes," he wrote, "no matter how normal, moral, or mature, one takes oneself to be."[45] While Laing's reading of the human condition is thoroughly Augustinian and Calvinistic, he has not accepted their solution of countering disease and death by choosing spiritual existence in Christ. Laing seems to agree with Luther that we are irresistibly sinful (*non posse non peccare*), but disagrees that grace can bring new existence simultaneous to the old (*simul peccator et iustus*).

Karl Menninger has argued from a more orthodox Reformed persuasion that we should abandon treating moral soul disorder as crime and see it in the therapeutic context. Where Laing, like Thomas Szass, is frightened by the use of medicine and psychiatry as societal sanction, both would agree with Menninger that "sins" such as prostitution, homosexuality, aggressive violence, and the like, should be decriminalized.[46] There is effective medical and psychiatric care for a wide variety of "moral" disorders and offenses, Menninger has suggested. To write off the criminal as a thoroughly evil person, who with clear mind and resolute intent aggresses and transgresses the well-being of himself and others, is to collapse the Pauline tension and expect persons to be univocally saint or sinner.

> The willfullness and the viciousness of offenders are part of the thing for which they have to be treated. They must not thwart our therapeutic attitude. It is simply not true that most of them are "fully aware" of what they are doing, nor is it true that they want no help from anyone, although some of them say so.[47]

Responding to the biblical truth that we live in a broken and rebellious cosmos, Laing quotes Kierkegaard five time in *The Divided Self*, arguing that we are inevitably a society bound to "sickness unto death." Mentally and morally sick individuals and families are merely "microsarcophagi" of this societal malaise.[48] What do we do? Let it go, counsels Laing. Perhaps the inherently human impulses will return if we diminish our moral and political pressure on persons. Here he accents a side of Calvin's anthropology that sees the original creation as a glory to God. Menninger, by contrast, has accented the fallenness and corruption of persons and their need of grace in the form of healing therapy. Both accent the poles of the Pauline antinomy. Menninger, the old Presbyterian elder from Kansas, counsels careful nurture, rigorous discipline, teaching, moral guidance, and comprehensive health care for those who fall into trouble. Laing says we don't need kindness but "mad liberation."[49]

This consideration of the health of the mind and madness or mental disease has been a cursory sketch of a profound and "yet to be explored" concern of both theology and psychiatry. It appears evident that soul health, mental health, and bodily health are intertwined. The nature of the interconnections and the identification of salutary preventive and interventive measures remains an exciting frontier of human knowledge.

Case Studies: Psychosurgery, Committal, Manipulation of Behavior

When we ponder the options before us of controlling and helping those who express the madness of the mind in terms of overt and societally offensive behavior, we come to three options: manipulation, isolation, and regeneration of the self. Psychosurgery has been tried, especially in the 1960s, for "pathologically aggressive behavior." Children in Mississippi who could not control their aggression and would not only harm others but continually bash their own heads against cement walls were operated on to burn out pathological focuses in their deep brains. John Doe, a psychosexual assailant in Michigan, was offered brain surgery (prefrontal lobotomy) to "cool down" his driving madness. Today such techniques are in some disrepute since we know so little about the structure and function of the brain, especially the exact action of surgical and chemical interventions. The Reformed tradition would not, I think, see surgery or even powerful chemotherapy as a long-range good in this field.

"Put them away forever! Don't let them near us!" This cry for imprisonment is strong from those who have seen madness acted out. But Menninger is right: punishment is a crime. It fosters greater crime, does not deal with the situation, and seldom brings healing or hope.

The same can be said for behavioral manipulation. While some habits can be cured by aversion therapy and the like, the majority of acted-out soul sicknesses will not respond to this modality of therapy. It, too, denies the freedom of reason and conscience and sees the human person more as a stimulus-response machine.

The therapies that will work are the experience of wholesome family life in childhood and the realistic coming to terms with the plight of the self in youth and adulthood. Knowing who we are as conflicted beings hell-bent on destruction of self and others in our fight against God but capable of grace and love in Christ's new humanity—this is the contribution of Christian faith to the realm of madness. We can discover the grace of interdependence and mutual aid as we acknowledge our need before God. Health is reconciliation and reciprocity with self, others, and God. Oneness is sanity.

Laing recalled Blake's poem: "The Angel that presided o'er my birth said: /Little creature, formed of joy and mirth/ Go, live without the help of anything on earth." Sad and true; but in a larger sense, wrong. The discovery that we have no help on earth is the "opening of paradise" (Luther). "Did we in our own strength confide, our striving would be losing." At the end of our rope, we bind ourselves to the "Galilean's side." Thankfully, God has seen that we also have much help on earth. The new being is fresh reminder of that deeply human commonality we share with each other, as well as the gracious undergirding of one another in *koinōnia*. Psychotherapy and psychoanalysis are gracious provisions in God's love—to help us clarify perceptions and deal a little better with reality (Freud).

Flannery O'Conner's story "A Good Man Is Hard to Find" depicted a madman's glimpse of himself. The "misfit" has just killed five members of an innocent family. He stands pathetically over the bleeding, dying grandmother.

> The misfit sneered slightly. "Nobody had nothing I wanted. . . . It was a head-doctor at the penitentiary said what I had done was kill my daddy but I known that for a lie. My daddy died in nineteen ought nineteen of the epidemic flu and I never had a thing to do with it. He was buried in the Mount Hopewell Baptist Church and you can go there and see for yourself.
>
> I found out the crime don't matter. You can do one thing or you can do another, kill a man or take a tire off his car, because sooner or later you're going to figger what it was you done and just be punished for it.
>
> The bleeding old lady found herself saying, "Jesus . . . Jesus" meaning, Jesus will help you. . . .
>
> "Yes'm," the misfit said as if he agreed. "Jesus thrown everything off balance. It was the same case with Him as with me except He hadn't committed any crime. . . . "Jesus was the only One that ever raised the dead," the misfit continued, "and He shouldn't have done it. He thrown everything off balance. If He did what He said, then it's nothing for you to do but throw away everything and follow Him, and if He didn't, then it's nothing for you to do but enjoy the few minutes you got left the best way

you can—by killing somebody or burning down his house or doing some other meanness to him. No pleasure but meanness."

      . . . "Maybe He didn't raise the dead," the old lady mumbled as she sank into the ditch.[50]

While we live, madness, being the "misfit," will be our lot. The resurrecting Jesus is to us life in our body of death. Disease, madness, and death are symptoms of the brokenness and incompleteness that mar our fallen existence. They are also signals of hope because they point to what we are becoming. "Our souls are restless," wrote Augustine, "until they rest in Thee."

·3·

Becoming Human:
Life's Transitions and Transactions

PASSAGES

The theme of passages, like that of suffering, could dominate our discussion of health and disease. This theme fascinates contemporary theologians, sociologists, and moralists, first, perhaps because the topic itself conveniently embraces the whole of human life from birth to death. Second, though, a scholar bold enough to tackle a study of the whole of human life may be himself caught in the most difficult "passage" of all, the middle years, a time when sensitive persons wrestle with fleeting time. Insight into life's mystery, its tenuousness, is not denied the young: witness the perception of Mozart, Marlowe, Pascal, Bonhoeffer. But an interpretive system as comprehensive as Erik Erikson's in *Childhood and Society*, for instance, assumes maturity, a storehouse of experiences painfully collected, patiently sifted, yielding finally an illuminating perspective on life's total fabric.

The word "passage" implies movement and direction. It implies, too, a story, of course, our story, our "narrative," as Dietrich Ritschl and others say. Even those who deny movement, direction, and purpose to the cosmos generally, and to the human story specifically, would not deny that the individual life has beginning, middle, and end. Medicine deals not only with crises at each stage of life, but with less easily diagnosed malaise all along the way, our "transactions" from one stage to another—say, from adolescence to young womanhood. Theology adds to this treatment a perception that life is not only a "chronological and developmental," but also a moral, movement. Our story inheres in "his" story, God's overarching will for human history.

"Passages" is a word laden with associations, particularly ethical ones. A theological view of passages will be elaborated shortly. Shakespeare's,

Erikson's, and Lawrence Kohlberg's analyses of passages are not overtly theological, yet they share with Reformed theology a common perception that passages imply choice, and price, and pain—that they are transacted in a moral universe, which assumes that some actions are "better" than others, that some relationships are "healthy" or "desirable" and others life-denying. Each of these systems, while it might purport only to describe what happens during the human being's life narrative, in fact fashions a normative model of what life could and should be.

The setting for each presentation is, again, tradition: that is, the social, moral, and historical context in which a life is lived. Shakespeare's vision of "healthy passages" must be gleaned from a total reading of the play in which the "all the world's a stage" speech occurs, for the cynical view of Jaques is, of course, precisely that negative life-bent which the playwright hopes to undercut through comedy. Man's "acts," Jaques intones, fall into "seven ages."

> At first the infant, mewling and puking in the nurse's arms,
> And then the whining school boy, with his satchel
> And shining morning faces, creeping like snail
> Unwilling to school. And then the lover,
> Sighing like furnace, with a woeful ballad
> Made to his mistress' eyebrow. Then a soldier
> Full of strange oath and bearded like the Pard
> Jealous in honor, sudden and quick in quarrel
> Seeking the bubble reputation
> Even in the cannon's mouth. And then the justice
> In fair round belly with good capon lined,
> With eyes severe and beard of formal cut,
> Full of wise saws and modern instances;
> And so he plays his part. The sixth age shifts
> Into the lean and slipper'd pantalloon,
> With spectacles on nose and pouch on side,
> His youthful hose well saved a world too wide
> For his shrunk shank; and his big manly voice,
> Turning again toward childish treble, pipes
> And whistles in his sound. Last scene of all,
> That ends this strange eventful history,
> In second childishness and mere oblivion,
> Sans teeth, sans eyes, sans taste, sans everything.[1]
> (*As You Like It*, II, vii, 143–66)

Jaques the cynic shares with Malvolio a "jakes" or privy vision of the human story. But as good comedy cuts through unbearable pretense (as we love to see the "bourgeois gentilhomme" or Tartuffe fooled at their own pretentious games), it also teases the grouch in us into a more "humane" perspective. Even though persons at all ages are foolish and ridiculous (What is more "ridiculous," i.e., laughable, than the sexual act? Yet life results from it.), we possess an indomitable will and a potential for joy and insight even in the midst of our pretense. So the "healthy minded" Rosalind, in this very play, chides the once ardent Orlando, who sighs "like a furnace,"

> Love is merely a madness, and . . . deserves as
> well a dark house and a whip as madmen do.
> (*As You Like It*, III, ii, 420–22)

She thereby defuses any expectation of tragic outcome the audience might have. So Olivia is "fooled" out of melancholy, Hal directed from riot or blood toward manhood, Lear baptized into self-giving, Prospero and Leonitas nudged toward forgiveness. Life moves through Jaques's seven stages, indeed, but need not sour or stagnate at any point. Jaques presents but one side of human possibility, the one perceived from the cynic's distance. Shakespeare presents us not so much with a stage but with a carnival in which we are participants and where joy, play, and affirmation are the order of the day.

Erikson, too, presents life's passages as seven stages, what he in *Young Man Luther* called "the metabolism of generations." Erikson contends that powers come into play at each stage to effect maturation or retardation. These powers are both intrinsic (i.e., intrapersonal and intrapsychic) and extrinsic (i.e., influenced by others, by circumstances and supervening grace, and by what Erikson might call fortune). "Each new being is received into a style of life prepared by tradition and held together by tradition, and at the same time disintegrating because of the very nature of tradition."[2] The fabric of tradition provides life a context and a foundation but the fabric is also torn and must be rewoven and extended to accommodate the new.

At each transition of life, Erikson writes, we are assisted toward the new task by the caring grace of significant others, including our community of belief and value, be it clan, village, family, or church. In the life crisis of early infancy the fondling of the mother grants "predictability and hopefulness to the baby's original chaos of urgent and bewildering body feelings."[3] In late infancy we are guided toward creative will, which overrides shame and doubt by others, particularly father and mother, as they allow for a healthy balance of rebellion and concession to imposed order. In childhood, psychosexual awareness emerges and one is aided toward affirmation and assertion despite omnipresent guilt, again by fantasy generated in association with parents and now peers. In school one learns through cooperation with others the delight of competency to understand things and make things work. Literacy, the power of shaping and being shaped by words, is developed. Here one discovers that when one asks and speaks, God and the universe speak and answer. As communicants we discover that we are *verantwortlich*, responsive and answerable. Finally, in the three adult identity crises one learns through reciprocity with others, through the transmission of life and value to children, and as one ages through gracious withdrawal into memory, hope, and contentment, the grace of accepting and letting go.[4]

Erikson's framework attests to the truth that a human life may as easily consume as elaborate itself. Some would argue that the general dispositional bent of a personality is set during the infancy stage, when "bonding" establishes a security that shapes all future development. Trust sustains, distrust sours, "healthy" development in Erikson's sense. Others insist that such a life-bent is genetically driven. Erikson does not seem to bow to such determinism, implying rather that choice (arising from moral freedom) confronts the individual at each stage. A person can foster or frustrate his own health (in any of the senses: physical, emotional, moral, and spiritual). The polarities Erikson presents have normative overtones:

Infancy	trust vs. mistrust
Early childhood	autonomy vs. shame and doubt
Play age	initiative vs. guilt
School age	industry and competence vs. helplessness
Adolescence	identity vs. alienation
Adulthood	intimacy, generativity vs. isolation, stagnation
Mature age	integrity and acceptance vs. resentment

Like Shakespeare, Erikson opts for life and relationship over death and alienation.[5] Lawrence Kohlberg has written of moral development as if it were a natural process, like biological and psychological development. If debility does not intervene, he says, we pass from stages of self-gratification to stages of mutuality and adherence to order to levels of higher justice, even altruism. This observation of physical and moral maturation in individual persons is then related to the belief that history, the human story itself, is also going somewhere. The valuation usually present is that we move from a present state to a better state. While chronological progress (aging) can hardly be denied, however, one might want to challenge Kohlberg's assumption that every, even many, individuals do indeed "progress" morally. Perhaps as readers and thinkers we shape our expectations too much by Sophocles, whose Oedipus Rex is driven (more accurately, drives himself) from a state of moral complacency into higher and higher levels of insight until he attains the final enlightenment with his symbolic self-blinding. As in *Lear*, we may feel that the insight is too dearly purchased, yet this model (that a person "ought" to grow away from narcissism into relation and finally toward universal enlightenment) is the one we favor. Tragedy and comedy alike move toward a Kohlberg-type vision, despite comedy's protests that it purports to present people as they are, not as they "ought" to be. Undoubtedly, many in Molière's audience, for instance, saw themselves reflected in M. Jourdain, "le bourgeois gentilhomme," and left the theater vowing they'd strut no more. But perhaps, too, the greater truth about human (moral) nature is that it does not "progress" very much away from Kohlberg's "stage one," in which M. Jourdain is frozen, or if it does, it does not grow very far, remaining as unenlightened as Molière's comic protagonist. Mutuality and justice are concepts ill-defined and poorly embraced, in this violent century as in any other. Pascal's thought that "the whole sequence of human beings, throughout the whole course of the ages, [is] the same man living on and learning something all the time"[6] may hold for scientific "learning" but hardly for moral behavior.

Passages in the Reformed Tradition

The Reformed tradition holds a double position: that progress is at best ambiguous, that development has a tragic underside.[7] Balancing this "realistic" anthropology, this awareness of the double nature of human personality, stands Christ, who increased in wisdom and stature and in divine as well as human favor (Luke 2:52, 4:21). This is the "normal" paradigm for growth and development in all its senses. Reformed theology is posited on the belief (present in Judeo-Christian tradition generally) that history is linear rather than cyclical, driving purposefully toward the end of time, when all will be made known. In this view, the underlying framework of history and the cosmos is moral and purposive even if the individual human life stagnates. God (to the Christian, God in Christ) provides the standard, God has set before us the way of life and of death. We are urged to choose life (Deut. 30:19). We develop morally across the life cycle if we receive at the right time the graces of the ability to know and love God, to esteem self, to respect and honor others, and to live with care on the earth. At every point of passage in our life we can go astray, but Jesus Christ, reflecting all of the Hebraic wisdom of God's leading into paths of righteousness (wholeness and rightness: Ps. 6, 23; Gen. 18:19), claims, "I am the way, the truth, and the life" (John 14:6).

This theological understanding of passages as being grounded in, and taking its standard from, God arises from the mists of ancient history. Hesiod, the father of Greek theology, regarded contemporary human sin, disease, misery, and death as a fall from a state of primal goodness. The *Theogony* (ca. 800 B.C.) presented the human saga as unfolding in the presence of the gods. *Weeks and Days*, written about the same time, recounted the creation of the five races of men and implied a similar falling away from some former state of health. The first race was the golden race, who knew no toil or sorrow. The earth abundantly served them; they did not age, but only fell asleep. These protohumans became angels (*daimones*), guardians of mortals. Second was the silver race, inferior in body and mind, who remained in perpetual childhood for one hundred years before their short and violent adult life. "They could not refrain from sinning one against the other, neither would they worship the deathless gods." These now dwell under the earth. Next, the bronze race perished by their own hands and now dwell in Hades. Fourth was the godlike race of hero-men, the demi-gods. Finally, in the present age of iron men, good is mingled with evil.

This degeneration of humankind, symbolized in *Weeks and Days* by a progression to baser metals, is analogous to what transpires in the individual soul. Torn between earth (finitude) and heaven (immortality), *elpis* (hope) was planted in the human soul (Pandora's box). Hope caused men both to "foresee their doom" and to hope for "cure from their diseases" (Aeschylus). Life thus understood as having divine origins and being measured against a transcendent standard would see itself and its world in terms of consequence, judgment, significance. Indeed, Hesiod viewed human life just so. The righteous transaction of the course of one's life, Hesiod believed, lies in working for justice. Work satiates hunger, fills the barn with livelihood, and pleases the gods. Justice is living peacefully and truthfully with one's fellows. Truthfulness, chastity, hospitality, and veneration of the aged are among the virtues commended within the scope of justice. Injustice in this world is punished by barren wives, poverty, disaster on land and sea. The just do "their work with gladness."[8]

For the ancients, life was of a piece, not only the world but all of one's life belonging to a pattern of meaning. Thus the passages of life were invested with great significance, as Joseph Fraser has illustrated in *The Golden Bough*. The rituals of incorporation into society, initiation into adulthood, and graduation to the seat of wisdom were imbued with sacral power, being moments when the gods touched persons' lives, drawing them into new vocations. Rites of passage such as that from adolescence into manhood clearly marked a movement, baptized it with meaning, and carried a freight of clearly understood obligations and expectations. The Jewish bar mitzvah or the Hopi Indians' coming-of-age rituals capture the intrinsic dignity of this passage of life more accurately than do the sentimental melodramas offered today on television. In these liturgical rituals or sacraments one becomes a leader of one's family and society. One becomes a warrior for God. The prolonged adolescence created by modern industrial society devastates natural adolescent growth because it refuses to accept what the young man or woman has already become. By contrast, life in earlier societies was a journey on a road with definite, predictable markers.

The Old Testament conception of life's passages as a journey with God originated with the historical journey of Abraham, who was believed to have been led by God out of Ur of the Chaldees. Israel's journey continued, with its infancy spent in Egypt, its youth addressed at Sinai, and its warrior-settlers led into the land of promise to experience stability and scattering, blessing and suffering, as a people come of age. This pilgrimage of Israel became the paradigm for movement in the course of one's personal life. When Tennyson wrote of life's consummate passage as "crossing the bar," or when the black slave sang "my home is over Jordan," this heritage was being recalled.

Our days pass away under the grace and wrath of God, as Psalm 90 expresses it. We are like wild desert grass that takes seed, sprouts, flowers dramatically, then shrivels, dies, and is blown away by the wind (v.6).

> Seventy years is the span of our life,
> Eighty if our strength holds,
> The hurrying years are labor and sorrow,
> So quickly they pass and are forgotten. (v.10)

Therefore, we "number our days" and apply our hearts unto wisdom (v. 12). The metaphor for human passages is organic: the growth, flourishing, and disintegration of the plant. The natural analogy complements the historical, in the Jewish understanding of life's passages. In Genesis 1:14, God said, "Let there be seasons." The Noachian covenant promised life "while seedtime and harvest endure" (Gen. 8:22). "For everything there is a season, a time to be born . . . a time to die" (Eccl. 1). Our life is measured into periods within a total span. Within these periods, framed by sufferings and blessings, appropriate duties emerge. In childhood one receives, in youth one learns, in adulthood one gives, in seniority one counsels and again receives (Heb. 5:13 ff.).

The New Testament likewise uses two analogues for the moral and spiritual transaction of life's passages. The first is the analogy of maturing faith. We are to develop greater maturity and assume greater responsibility as we grow up. We are milk-fed in the days before we are accountable. Then we move on to solid food, at which stage we discern good and evil (Heb. 5:13). Pictures of natural things being planted, growing, maturing, and becoming fruitful punctuate the Gospels and Epistles (Luke 8:15; Matt. 13:26; John 15:2; Rom. 7:4). The image is twofold. On the one hand there is a natural unfolding and development, a springing forth, that is necessary because of the fruitful creativity of God, the ground of being. Secondly, there is an emphasis on deliberate choice and careful gardening and watering. We must nurture life toward its possibility against the threat of retarding and destructive forces (Mark 4:20 ff.).

The New Testament paradigm for healthy human development is, as has been stated, Christ's story. His nativity amid both peaceful, silent wonder and violent terror (with the slaughter of the innocents) prefigures our own violent yet miraculous birth. Then, appearing in the temple and interpreting the Torah, he dignified the passage of life from adolescence into young manhood, as he assumed moral leadership. Christ the teacher demonstrated in receiving little children the blending of strength and gentleness, "wise as a serpent, gentle as a dove," a wisdom that recognized the child's joy and wonder at life as the right vision: "of such is the kingdom of God" (Mark 10:15; Luke 18:17).

As Christ died unjustly a young man, God's sacrifice of himself to human will, we, too, must come of age. We must begin to witness to truth and right even when the world around us hates and tries hard to extinguish such light. We call to ourselves the antagonism and enmity of the world. Maturing existence in God is cruciform (Matt. 16:24; Gal. 2:20). It suffers, it pays the price for advancing the world from where it is to the new place where it should be. As Pannenberg has written: "The kingdom of God confronts the world at every turn as its own future."[9] The world prefers the old, the established, the status quo. The young person who lives prophetically, that is, responsive to God's voice and moral will, brings judgment to this orientation and pain upon himself.

The serenity of maturity and the contentment of the person near death is like the resurrection. Here we know that just as the world cannot save and heal, the world cannot harm or kill. At this passage we know that power lies elsewhere, that the Lord gives and takes away (Job 1:21), that since he is with us in the valley of death no evil is to be feared (Ps. 23). Here with Christ we commend life for its final passage into his hands (Luke 23:46).

The main import of the Christian Gospel on life's passages is not in the lessons we draw from Christ's life as we follow "in his steps" but in the career of Jesus as he fashioned new being in the bosom of humanity (2 Cor. 5:17). We recognize God as ruler because the kingdom of Christ has been established as the future horizon of this world. God is establishing his reign, his lordship, in the creation. The life, death, and resurrection of Jesus and the decisive, unprecedented, and unrepeated moment of power in the primitive apostolic community is the inauguration of this new order, new reality, new being. From that moment on, political authority, human accomplishment, and personal passage into maturity come only "from above" (John 19:11). Jesus announced that the kingdom was near as persons were being healed, became whole, discovered themselves, and came to understand all that they were and were to be (John 4:6 ff.). In the Gospel miracles, healings, and encounters with the Lord, a new reality was introduced that became a fresh context for life's pilgrimage. Christ's new community is made up of those who have been claimed by his future. Their life story now becomes the narrative of his rule.

"Our times are in thy hands." The doctrine of providence and predestination in our life's course arrived at its full development in the work of Augustine. In contrast to the Pelagians, who thought of human development and maturation in terms of creative assertion, achievement, and edifying action, Augustine emphasized the guidance of God into crises of challenge, through such crises in confidence of God's faithful companionship, and out the other side, tested yet victorious. "Our thoughts and words [are] in the hand of God," Augustine wrote. Problems that appear on that path are to be boldly "approached and solved."[10]

Calvin continued this tradition by speaking of the Lord's calling as the basis of "our way of life" (*Institutes*, 3.10.6, p. 724). Our calling is both constraint and challenge. It limits the range of free choice about who we are and what we do, yet it is the vehicle for the fulfillment of our being and action. Our calling is mediated through our parents; our homes; the activation of our gifts in education and community; the work we choose; domestic, civil, and ecclesial associations; and the personal way we confront life's challenges and sufferings. "Lest in our stupidity and rashness everything be turned topsy-turvey [*omnia sursum deorsum miscerentur*], he has appointed duties for every man in his particular way of life" (p. 724). Harmony is discovered "among the several parts of life" when it is ordered to the divine goal of the Lord's calling.

> Forgetting what is behind me, and reaching out for what lies ahead, I press towards the goal to win the prize which is God's call to [onward and upward] life in Christ Jesus. (Phil. 3:14, my translation)

The call of God is the voice on the horizon that beckons us along life's paths, where each moment becomes a particular opportunity to glorify God.

As we move into the post-Reformation phase of Calvinist thought we find in Puritanism and Protestant orthodoxy a tendency so to regularize and allegorize the human pilgrimage that it becomes a static phenomenon. Life's journey is not, after all, a predictable, abstract set of events, each one reducible to markers on a spiritual map. *Everyman* startles the reader with its presentation of our final hours. *Pilgrim's Progress* leans on exact equations (each step of life is but a symbol of one stage of our spiritual quest). Marlowe's Dr. Faustus and Shakespeare's Hamlet (and, indeed, most of the Shakespearean heroes) capture more realistically the sense articulated through the Old and the New Testament—that the journey follows no secure path but is fraught throughout with hazards, detours, surprises: such, after all, are the consequences of human freedom. Dr. Faustus, we admit, was a "good" man (we might label him as "Type A, Obsessive-Compulsive") who envisioned, sought, and achieved a worthy goal: the acquisition of knowledge. Free choice, as powerful a gift as rationality or feeling, alters the great man's itinerary, and reverses, rather than advances, the "smooth transition" of his life's passages.

Two themes in the Westminster Confession of Faith (1646) illustrate the orthodox Protestant understanding of life's passages. On the one hand, God, the transcendent, unchanging sovereign, stands over the exigencies of our existence, reducing them to transitory insignificance. "God, infinite in being and perfection . . . works all things according to the counsel of his own immutable and most righteous will."[11] Another emphasis points to the freedom and spontaneity in God and in human action: "Although God knows whatsoever may or can come to pass upon all supposed conditions, yet hath he not decreed anything because he foresaw it as future, or as that which would come to pass upon certain conditions" (3.2, p. 198).

In that age, as in all before it, when plagues devastated young lives and premature death was the norm, the divine regulations of life's movements were highlighted and attention was focused on God's constant care and judgment, drawing all persons to repentance through the crises of life. The septicemia crises of childhood or the pneumonic crises of young adulthood were occasions for divine confrontation. In Puritan New England, for example, Cotton Mather considered the sickbed as the God-given opportunity to apprise persons of their end and of Christ's proffered salvation.[12] As the Puritan preachers reflected on life's treacherous course, they saw that only the enduring promises and covenant of grace could sustain people on their journey.

> In the covenant of grace: wherein he freely offered unto sinners life and
> salvation by Jesus Christ, requiring of them faith in him that they may be
> saved, and promising to give unto all those that are ordained unto life his
> Holy Spirit, to make them willing and able to believe. (7.3, p. 202)

Nineteenth- and twentieth-century Reformed thought has accented the relationship between God and people in the covenant of grace. This has had distinctive meanings for the covenant of life and the course of life. Schleiermacher, in the spirit of Calvin, claimed that we could not say much about the divine essence but could speak only of the manifestation of God's relation to us in the experiences of life. Moments of grand and awful experience and of simple delights are moments when we are conscious of ultimacy, when we are known by God. These moments deepen life; in personal fulfillment we gain some sense of the meaning, character, and momentum of our life.[13]

Karl Barth wrote of the intersection of God's light and word into space and time as witnessed in our allotment of life. Time is the divinely given space for human life. "God gives us time, and we have it, as we need it for life and may actually have it for this purpose—no more and no less" (*Dogmatics*, III/2, p. 554). Here we have Calvin's doctrine of the predestined human story and the Puritan notion of the decree and ordination of those measures of life. Life under God is distinguished not by its duration but by its depth. We are not to begrudge life's brevity, not to bemoan its passing, not to "accept our allotment of time," but to "welcome it with gratitude and joy" (p. 555). Human life, while impressive as an unfolding story, is also miraculous in the unfathomable and inexhaustible depth that the vertical relation to the Creator bestows. Even a short life can be full of power, beauty, and lasting significance. The long life can be boring and of little use to God or anyone else. "Man belongs to God and to his fellows." God seems to "fling at man" a twofold taunt: "Once you were not!" and "One day you will be no more." "Will you at this time restore the kingdom?" Jesus was asked. "It is not for you to know about dates or times, which the Father has set within his own control"(Acts 1:7-8). As the Psalmist counseled, we best live between the times in devotion and service, for life's measure and meaning ultimately remain a mystery. The presence of God liberates us in this allotment of life. We are emancipated from the transiency and bondage of life; in creative faith, love, and hope, our time becomes no longer *chronos* but *kairos* (Gal. 4:4).

Case Study: The Conquest of Aging

Many bioethical problems facing us today deal with the issue of fulfilling, negating, or modifying what we have identified as the passage points along the life cycle: intervening in infancy, latency, or adolescence; amending human parenting and the transmission of life; manipulating human structure in adult change of life; effecting change in aging and dying. Many of the ethical quandries of biomedicine pertain to the attempts to technologize, morally relativize, or manipulate the passages of life. Birth and infancy as well as dying are increasingly viewed as clinical phenomena.

But human beings can't be reduced to data: that basic truth which Victor Hugo and Charles Dickens so emphasized in the nineteenth century holds even more today. David, the Houston bubble baby, grew according to biological charts, but yet might have died had the medical staff not realized that he needed to be touched. The healthy baby monkey given a wire mother and a bottle will die. That Dickens's Paul Dombey survives past infancy, deprived first of his mother, then of his nurturing housemaid, is due only to his loving sister. Human beings cry out at all ages for relation, warmth, affirmation, even when they enjoy the wonders of modern technology.

Many of the crises that arise during life's turning points issue from needs that lie deeper than pills can reach. Substitution therapies, perhaps smoking, excessive drinking, or drugs, not only fail to cure the malaise but may arrest healthy physical and emotional maturation. (At twenty-one, a young alcoholic in one case study exhibited the emotional reactions of a fourteen-year-old: those years had been literally "lost," his mother observed.) The much discussed condition anorexia nervosa may both begin with and lead to unhealthy self-obsession. As Hilda Bruch has written, an anorexic may view herself as so offensive to God that constant fasting and purgation are required. As a result of this pathological belief (concentration on demand rather than on grace), self-perception is distorted and relationships are disturbed, for one feels disgusting in the presence of others. Because the primary relationship with God is out of focus, love for self and others has become distorted. A new series of studies compares anorexia with the obsessive devotion to running and other exercises exhibited by many middle-aged men. Like anorexics, the researchers say, runners may suffer from an identity crisis.

> In both runners and anorexics, the running and dieting start at a testing time in life. . . . Many men face their most vulnerable time in life when gradually declining physical prowess coincides with possible career and

> sexual disappointments. Some . . . hope to set their lives to rights by
> fanatical dedication to running.[14]

The key phrase for understanding these disturbances may be "grace rather
than works." But therein lies the mystery: grace must be received; it cannot be won. And it cannot be manufactured in the laboratory.

We tend to "medicalize" and "demoralize" each of the transitions in
life's passages. Childhood anxiety may be treated by Ritilin rather than by
careful health instruction and changed parenting patterns. Birth control
devices are dispensed alongside the junk-food machines, thus avoiding for
adults the strain and shame of discussing sex and sexual mores with our
adolescents. Pregnancy, menopause, and their male counterparts are seen
as objects of pharmacologic and psychologic therapy. The challenge to im-
bue these transitions with healing and saving blessing remains; the new
generation senses this deprivation of ritual and communal definition and
benediction for life's passages. Their flight to highly disciplined cults, to
natural foods, or to therapy groups reflects a yearning for renewed spiritual-
moral celebration of life's passages.

Ivan Illich remains the critic of this medicalizing, which he views as
another form of consumerism, robbing persons of their ability to care for
themselves. Into Mexican villages, Illich writes,

> where life passages have been dealt with in traditional and comforting
> ways, have come the nurse and doctor, teaching the people about an evil
> pantheon of clinical deaths, each one of which can be banned, at a price.
> Instead of modernizing people's skills for self-care, they preach the ideal
> of hospital death. By their ministration they urge the peasants to an un-
> ending search for the good death of international description, a search
> that will keep them consumers forever.[15]

No one would want to return to the preantibiotic age. But neither independence nor interdependence should be sacrificed to a sterile goal of "scientific progress."

Technically, aging begins at the moment of conception. Usually, however, the term designates the transition through the last of life's passages.
Is aging a disease? The United States government has established The National Institute on Aging with the equivocal purposes of securing greater
health as we grow older and investigating the causes of and solutions for
the aging process. As we grow older, certain little-understood, genetically driven biological mechanisms come into play to diminish vigor, increase susceptibility to disease, and compromise the viability of tissues

and organs. Most biologists (e.g., Fries, Stanford) feel that there is a built-in "biological clock" and a "natural life span" that render our life history an arc or trajectory as opposed to an ascent or descent interrupted by morbid and mortal assaults. Proposals now abound to examine the mechanisms of this process and to slow them down. The social and political effects of these proposals are widely discussed and highly controversial. How might the Reformed ethical tradition respond to this development?

Initially, the tradition would concur with the desire to understand disease and to remove the causes of premature death. Diseases, hormonal aberrations, or toxic assaults that lead to premature death should be the object of our ethical concern, just as John Wesley and the religious reformers of the nineteenth century sought to alleviate the industrial conditions (e.g., child labor) that brought about premature and unnatural death. Disorders, in other words, that are brought on by our stupidity, malice, and greed are inimical to the good life that God intends for his children.

In the second place, the Reformed tradition would initiate and support efforts to enhance the human life span. Our vocation, our calling to pilgrimage, to cocreative labor with God in the world, is enhanced by a long and healthy life. We are obliged to safeguard the length of this life in ourselves and in others. The efforts to prevent and cure disorders that cut life short before its promise is fulfilled are well and good, symbolic of our resistance to evil and our anticipation of the kingdom. To live to be ninety, and to transact the passages of toiling young adult, contented older adult, and wise-fool octogenarian, is indeed a divine blessing.

Finally, however, the church should resist efforts to extend indefinitely the human life span; to freeze dead bodies, hoping for resuscitation when a medical cure is found for that vector of death; and to radically eliminate the aging process. Responding to the faith principles of celebration of living and dying in the divine provision of a life's course, of finitude as a condition of our humanity, and of the beneficence of passing on the power of existence to succeeding generations, we should accept aging and death as inevitable events comprehended in life's mystery.

The means toward such acceptance are perhaps a trust in the evident provisions of God, combined with a healthy self-esteem that anticipates and rises to meet change. But acceptance, grace, and wisdom are painfully won, not only in advanced age but at every stage. The resistance and the release, in fact the central human anguish of "passages," has been captured in the haunting harmonies of Richard Strauss and the poignant lyrics of Hugo von Hofmannsthal in *Der Rosenkavalier*. Audience and singers have been caught in a time warp, with time suspended through the affec-

tion expressed between the Marshallin and her young lover, Count Octa-
vian. Although she has found in the young man all the warmth her starved
heart had craved, and desires to prolong this ecstasy (and her own fading
youth), she surrenders him to a sweetheart his own age. Hers is the dilemma of the middle years: when desires and perspectives are fresh but neither
wisdom nor patience have arrived to sustain collapse. "Half a life away"
she had been an expectant young girl, but in the irony of passages the experience that has seasoned her naiveté with depth has robbed her of years.
Strauss's concluding trio captures the grace of her yielding to time but does
not gloss over her pain. She suffers intensely, yet life continues.

Each passage of life is a threshold where our life is opened to new possibility. Each is crisis in the biblical sense: a breaking in of divine power and
demonic threat. If the soil that sustains the plant is rich and firm, if the
ingredients of sun, rain, and nutrients are present, the flower blossoms, the
metamorphosis occurs, and a new form of this particular entity, long and
arduously prepared by God through nature, is given to the world.

SEXUALITY

> So God created man in his own image; in the image of God he created
> him; male and female he created them . . . . (Gen. 1:27)

Sex sells. It also confounds, delights, tortures, and soothes the least and
the greatest of us, for no human lacks a sexual component in his general
makeup. Old women become young and wise men become fools before
sexual devastations, as comedy has long depicted. The shaft of Cupid's ar-
row can turn a dignified statesman into a babbling idiot. And as Freud
taught us, infancy is no paradise, old age is no protection, and even family
relationship is no guarantee against sexual feelings.

Thus sexuality (its nature and its crises) weaves its way through the
passages of our lives, raising in particular the moral questions so often considered in general. Platonic detachment does not fit well with actual experience: persons matter, affections matter, feelings intrude. The touching
that La Leche mothers say babies need for their emotional health is craved
by all of us at all stages of our life. When, and with whom, that touching is
to be found creates the grand drama—too often, the bitter tragedy—of
each life.

Sexuality is not a one-dimensional phenomenon, nor a two-headed mon-
ster of the Dr. Jekyll/Mr. Hyde type. Sexual morality might be defined as
"whatever is pleasing is permitted," and yet that pleasure yields a bitter

fruit: abortion, disease, unexpected emotional entanglements, sex without love. But a stricter view of sexual morality may also bring harm: overpopulation, double standard, undue obsession with sex, sex without love.

Sex, often described as "the beast with two backs," simply does not fit into a comfortable classification and "sexuality" (that is, total sexual being, including a whole range of noncoital physical and emotional needs, such as touching) defies analysis. Language, too, often confuses: where the Greeks deployed an arsenal of words in an effort to pin down sexuality (eros, agape, and the like), an American says equally, "I like pizza," "I love pizza," and "I love my boyfriend." A Frenchman or a German lacks even "like" to express milder emotion, being stuck with *aimer* and *lieben* to cover clothes, culture, grandparents, and lovers.

When one leaves general discussion for particular cases, sexuality appears to belong to some moral sphere of its own, particularly as one attempts to balance competing "goods." Sexual infractions—condemned in the Bible along with stealing and killing—pale alongside of the manufacture of nuclear weapons or the Auschwitz atrocities. Jesus dispersed the howling mob ready to stone the adulterous woman (where was her partner?) by reminding the men of their own complicity in sexual sin. Yet the fury remains, framed in the American consciousness as the image of Hester Prynne standing on the scaffold with "A" on her bosom, or the law in Iran that today punishes sexual "crime" by death. Sleeping with one's lover is sanctioned in some cultures, frowned on in others, forbidden in many. Sexual attitudes shift with time and place but always remain persistently in the forefront, a concern for "moral purity" (again, necessarily scantily defined) often outstripping a concern for keeping our planet in one piece. Even admitting that "none is good save God alone," people (particularly women) are often stamped "good" or "bad," not on the basis of their reverence for human life, their affection for friends or family, or their devotion to God, but to the degree to which they keep their sexuality within conventionally prescribed bounds.

So entangled do our ideas about sexuality remain that we retain this moral obsession (understandable in dualistic cultures, where the body was denounced in order to favor the mind) alongside of a parallel tendency to pretend that sex is no more than a biological function, like respiring, defecating, or masticating. We don't make love, we copulate. Procreation, rather than being seen as a natural issue of sexual union, has been joined with technology, from sperm banks to in vitro fertilization. Abortion and birth-control devices (including the pocket full of rubbers) further confuse matters. But experience shows that sexuality refuses to be reduced to the mechanical as persistently as it refuses to yield to manageable ethical cate-gories. Sexuality, not just sexual excitement, reaches into our deepest self and makes us tremble. "I can't get no satisfaction," Mick Jagger has been complaining for twenty years, referring not so much to failed orgasm but to the whole set of intimate physical, emotional, and spiritual needs we possess in common.

Sexuality in the Reformed Tradition

It is exactly because of this penetration of sexuality into all corners of our life that religious systems persistently have worried over it. Many research-ers have pointed to certain sexual ideas and taboos, such as incest, held in common across cultures and centuries, as indicating the existence of uni-versal or normatively "human" standards of sexual behavior. Among these prohibitions (always stronger than recommendations) the common de-nominator seems to be that inversion (narcissism, violence, lack of regard for the partner as a "thou") is condemned, and relation (self-giving, recep-tivity, reciprocity) is praised. Invasion sours and spoils life; relation sweetens and enriches it. Simply stated, sexual behaviors that could be seen as interrupting individual or community well-being would be dis-couraged. "Healthy," "normal," and, therefore, "moral" sexual activity would be that which creates the family, nurtures children, enables both man and woman to fulfill their social tasks, and fosters in both sexes con-tentment and hope.

But religious systems, the Reformed among them, have seen sexuality as more than social cement, more than personal palliative. Sexuality is an essential quality of the divine engagement with the human. The Genesis passage reveals that God's image is conveyed into human life through the man-woman being together. Not only is a child, *imago dei*, created by that act, but the act itself represents "knowing." We know and we are known as God interacts with his creation.

Human intimacy and fidelity display God within our existence. To "know" one another in sexual intercourse is to know God (Isa. 11:2; Jer. 22:16; Hos. 4:1,6). It is also to know bliss and terror, for it is to know good and evil—hence the connection with the tree in the garden. The paradise narratives are cast in sexual imagery, showing that God desired friendship in creating people (Gen. 2:5) and that man's fulfillment required a partner (Gen. 2:18–25).

Sexuality, then, was inextricably bound up with the Hebrew under-standing of God's relation to his world. To be fruitful and multiply was a divine mandate as well as a blessing. Fertility and procreative power were benedictions on lives that had found favor with God (Ps. 127:5; Gen. 17:2). The purpose of the sexual life was to perpetuate the divine family and glorify God's name. The misdirections of this purpose—masturbation, prostitution, homosexuality, bestiality, sodomy, and adultery—were severely condemned. In contrast to the orgiastic religion of Canaanite Baalism and the other neighboring fertility religions, a strict code of family fidelity and chastity was imposed on the covenant. Sex was neither denigrated nor glorified. These two deviant tendencies were constantly checked by the Hebrew reading of God's will. The longing of woman and man for each other was natural and good; and to companionship was added delight as one of the gifts of intimacy (Cant. 1:9).

Of course, "couples" did not remain long in this paradisiacal state. "In Adam's Fall we sinned all," as an old copy book has it: the curse of "knowing" accompanied the blessing. Man toiled, woman anguished in childbirth. Hence, sexual "rules" have always sat alongside the ideal of healthy God-reflecting sexuality.

In the Talmud we are told that God's people, Israel, received from Yahweh in the time of Noah a universal law, a *jus gentium*, a natural law, that applied to all people. This was not the more demanding and particular Mosaic Code, which made special requirements on the nation Israel; this law, which the Hebrews called Noachian law, applied to all persons. In addition to respect for the Lord only, for his name, for civil authority, for life in other persons and animals, Noachian tradition contended that we respect and fulfill the self and another before God by man-woman fidelity, which receives generate life as the gift of God's hand (hence the sanctions against fornication, adultery, homosexuality, and other forms of inversion or perversion). It also proscribed abortion. We can assume from the force of the prohibition that these diversions from natural and holy patterns of sexual expression were widespread.

Sexual health, like well-being generally, is an available but elusive state. We tend to be well and do well in the sexual sphere if nature's patterns and rhythms are gracefully received. If we despise the natural and try too hard to create something extraordinary, sexuality can become a hightly destructive force. Maintaining the balance between accepting boundaries on the one hand and correcting "flaws" or creating the novel on the other is essential in sexual ethics. The covenant code, the holiness code, and other moral texts in the Hebrew Scriptures amplified and elaborated these basic Noachian values.

The New Testament continues this tradition of celebrating the life of the body, marriage, and the family. Jesus' teaching (Matt. 19:4–9) and

Pauline instruction (Eph. 5:25, 28) sustain the emphasis on the goodness and necessity of sexuality and marital life. But another note is added: the New Testament, expecting apocalyptically the end of time, and reflecting the asceticism of the Essenes (Qumran), as well as a dualism between spirit and flesh (influenced here by the Persians), cautions against undue concentration on this world, this body, sex, even the procreative orders of marriage and family. According to this view, lust of the flesh is a diverting energy, turning us away from our true devotion to God's kingdom and its righteousness (Matt. 5:28; Rom. 13:14). Passion misdirected into sexual lust is idolatry. In place of the divine image, which is to constitute the radiance of love, we constitute an idol, a penultimate image and likeness. We worship another form and attraction.

The Christian Gospel brought to the world a new answer for the wholeness of persons. Salvation (*sōtēria*) is a quality of being wherein one is rescued from allurements that lead *out* of life, toward illusion and seduction and death, for fulfillment *in* life. As such, it is concerned not only for the quality, but for the fruits, of sexual liaison. Christian moral scrutiny involved not only acts in themselves but the intentions within such acts as well as the results of actions. The seeds of deontologic, characterologic, and utilitarian ethics are found in the Gospel. The issues that sexual ethics have concerned itself with have to do both with what happens to the persons involved and with the issue of the relationship. The total health of one and all, within oneself, between selves and God, between selves and other selves, was now a paramount, some say an obsessive, concern of Christian ethics.

The primitive Christian community, guided by Paul, Peter, and the other apostles, adhered strenuously to a Christian version of Jewish sexual doctrine, adding the strictures of bodily chastity as found in apocalyptic Judaism (such as that of the Qumran community on the shores of the Dead Sea). Jesus lived and taught these precepts, loving, as every good Jew did, the body, the joy of human friendship, and the goodness of creation.

As the Lord's spirit established and sustained the fragile Christian community within the Roman Empire, this sense of sexual responsibility intensified spiritually and was soon codified into formal rules. The life, death, resurrection, and living spiritual companionship of Christ with the primitive church had chastened the phenomenon of love with a new depth. *Phileō*, the respectful and tender friendship of Greek culture, now became *agapē*, the mysterious self-giving, unqualified concern for the other. In the *Didache*, two ways were seen to lie before us: the way of life and the way of death. The way of life is *agapē*, pure love for God, self, and others. We are to abstain from bodily lusts and practice nonretaliation and forgiveness. Similarly, we must refrain from the common pagan practices of corrupting youth, adultery, prostitution, aborting fetuses, and exposing newborns.[16] Whereas pagans, with the blessing of their philosophers (Plato's *Republic*, 5.461; Aristotle's *Politics*, 7.16), widely practiced abortion for reasons ranging from concealing adultery, maintaining feminine beauty, dividing patrimony, and controlling population, the Christian honors life more respectfully since the fruit of sexual union is the divine gift.[17]

In A.D. 309 bishops and presbyters traveled to the town of Granada, in Spain, to formulate in eighty-one sentences the earliest extant canons of Christian behavior. Almost half of the statements referred to human sexual conduct. Like the Noachian formulations, a great proportion of this instruction dealt with *moicheia*: sexual misconduct. The synod spelled out in detail the spiritually and morally damning power of adultery, divorce, fornication, prostitution, homosexuality, abortion, pornography, and public spectacles that abused the sacred dignity of human sexual love. (Later, Puritan antipathy to plays and dances stemmed from the same belief that the sacred dignity of sexuality should not be desecrated.)

Amid the alarm and condemnation expressed in these great moral teachings, proferring of repentance and restitution can also be found. Elvira Canon 31, for example, reads:

> Young men who after the faith of saving baptism have committed sexual offense shall be admitted to communion when they marry, provided the required penance is done....[18]

As early as the second century, Jewish-Christian faith portrayed elements that would be continued in the medieval, Reformation and Puritan-Presbyterian theology of human sexuality: a vision of human fulfillment and faithfulness in the chaste life, fidelity in marriage, and the respectful receiving of children as the gifts of God.

Augustine elaborated a Christian view of human sexuality in its divine prospect as well as its demoniac potential. The heart of his theology of sexuality, which influenced all subsequent Western thought, focused on the pervasiveness of misdirected desire: concupiscence, or lust. We find in ourselves, he wrote, a ravenous appetite to be something we are not and to possess what is not our own. The primal transgression, eating the apple from the tree of knowledge, mingled in one image appetite (hunger and desire) with sexuality (hunger, desire, and "knowing") and morality (all these plus designation of good and evil). But for our banishment from

Eden, he said, we would have grasped the secret of mortality and complete life. For Augustine, happiness consisted of contentment with what one has and wanting only that to which one has a right. Dissatisfied with this, humans have found themselves with an unbridled, insatiable craving. The assault was on the fount of life and on pleasure itself. The assault is not only against God; it is against ourselves. Dissatisfied with our divinely established nature (*ab ipso esse*), we impose a variant will that hurts not God, but ourselves (*C.D.* 12.3). The image of his being within us cannot be injured; we can only degrade ourselves by our antagonism to his will and lead ourselves body and soul into restless torment. The result is perpetual restlessness that is satisfied only when the heart again finds its true home.

The condition of misdirected will is inherited and organic. If Augustine had possessed modern knowledge, he might have said that sin was genetically determined. Not only are sin and guilt transferred biologically as parents transmit life to their children, but the sexual acts of intercourse, conception, gestation, and birth themselves are sinful. The organs of sexuality and the sexual act are the transmitters of corruption from generation to generation: " . . . all of these evils, some fifty, from ambition to unchastity, including some too filthy to be named, arise out of the root of that error and perverse affection which every son of Adam brings into the world with him" (*C.D.* 22.22).

Augustine seems to imply (here agreeing with Tertullian and other Latin fathers) that both coitus and procreation would have been autonomous functions, like breathing and hearing, had man not sinned and ruined paradise (*C.D.* 14.24). Now, said these theologians, sex and the sex organs are shrouded in shame.

Sexual desire and sexual activity, then, are symptomatic of man's general degradation. But is sex a life dimension that was once good, and is even now fundamentally good, or is it redeemed only in grace? Augustine does allow (though briefly and reluctantly) for marriage constrained by Jesus' recapitulation of the Mosaic blessing: "Have you not read—at the beginning God made them male and female—therefore a man shall leave his father and cleave unto his wife." He also emphasizes Paul's instruction for husbands to love their wives (*C.D.* 14.24). Augustine gives fuller development to the issues of sexuality and marriage elsewhere in his writings and admits in his *Retractions* that he has not satisfactorily dealt with the subject. Yet to our benefit he has emphasized that sexuality, like other energies, can be, and, indeed, is, a distraction from God and from one's true self. Sexuality can become the joining of oneself to an alien body substituted for one's intended love, God.

The Augustinian vision safeguards the high purpose and special dignity of human sexuality. The danger of his position, however, lies in the subtle denigration of even the wholesome and generative expressions of sexuality. It does this by surrounding sex itself with an aura of suspicion and guilt and subordinating it to a status inferior to that of celibacy.

Augustine, then, elaborated on the double view toward sexuality found within the Scriptures themselves, identifying the universal shame over, and uneasiness about, our sexuality with our falling away from goodness. Primitive taboos, caustic stipulations of the first high religions, and Greek and Roman comedies had hovered nervously around the subject, as though there were something inherently ridiculous about sexual needs. Augustine gathered their universal psychology into one grand theological vision of human life. He pointed to Christ's freedom and salvation as offering release from the underlying disease, alienation from God, and its symptoms, self-obsession, guilt, and pride. Furthermore, although Augustine articulated an understanding of sexuality that was to be embodied in societal and ecclesial tradition (the world of *civitas terrena*), he also announced freedom from such constraint in *civitas dei*, which transcends the city of man and offers liberated citizenship. Now sexuality could move into the status of *adiaphoroa*, of things morally neutral, even into the thoughtless contemporary "freedom" that threatens to become a new bondage. Augustine's perspective on sexuality placed the moral issues of sexual practice and the transmission of life into a framework wherein the Reformers could speak of marriage and generation as vocation.

Paul and Augustine claimed that human freedom is threatened by two deviations: law and flesh. Calvinism and Puritanism have leaned toward the legalistic distortion. Following Calvin's successor Theordore Beza, the English and American Calvinist Puritans developed a morálism that became the foundation of Victorian sexual repression and hypocrisy. Calvin himself, however, maintained the vibrant dialectic wherein freedom did not collapse into either legalism or libertarianism.

Calvin's theology of sexual behavior is encapsuled in his exposition of the seventh commandment:

> Because God loves modesty and purity, all uncleanness must be far from us. To sum up, then: we should not become defiled with any filth or lustful intemperance of the flesh. (*Institutes*, 2.8, p. 405)

This somber passage, extolling conventional and temperate morality, shows the preference of the Calvinist tradition for order and moderation, leaning into the vice of formalism as Luther leaned toward license. Augustine's experienced counsel to shun the allurements of erotic desire and sublimate those same powerful energies into *amor dei* became the counsel of frugality and ascetic discipline. Courtship, marriage, and the bearing and rearing of children were now seen as vocation. Marriage, no longer the allowance of Paul or the concession of Augustine, became the verifying expression of salvation and the vehicle for good work in the world. Sexuality and marriage took on economic virtue. The positive meaning of the commandment, Calvin believed, was that we "chastely and continently regulate all parts of our life" (*Institutes*, p. 405). Marriage and childbearing were seen as divinely instituted blessings and duties. Extramarital, nonconjugal liaisons of any kind were proscribed because they were both illicit and unproductive. Marriage, safeguarding chastity, allowed the divine work to proceed in and through us. Modesty, in Calvin's splendid phrase, was "purity of heart joined with chastity of body" (*Institutes*, p. 407).

Sexual morality, then, is linked in Calvin's system with both conscience and Christian vocation. Persons are encouraged to discern the particular will of God for them in their way and walk of life. Here we meet one of the most powerful moral doctrines in the Western tradition: the notion that there is a particular destiny for each person, a peculiar divine imperative in every situation. Conscience, that intimate knowledge of God's will, personally imparts this calling and this judgment. Furthermore, Calvin continued, chastity in individuals is tested if the thought and speech of the culture is sordid. Provocation and pornography at the societal level are to be lamented as much as is personal indiscretion.

Calvin's view of sexuality conveys the bilateral temperament that we noted in the Reformed estimate of well-being. We are living here and now in our bodies, and as good stewards we carefully manage them. We are not our bodies, as the current liberation school would argue, but rather our body is a vessel of the divine spirit. This world is not all there is. Yet we do not escape the body or the world; rather, we bring the body under the discipline of what Max Weber called the "inner worldly asceticism." This paradoxical spirit of negation and affirmation led the Calvinist to esteem marriage highly, to avoid moral degradation, and to assume rigorous responsibility in procreation and parenting. Marriage, sexual purity, and family life were not regarded as ultimate ends in themselves, however. Rather, they instrumentally served to purify the soul and, second, to cooperate with God in his redemptive building of the world.

Puritanism is as little understood as Calvinism, particularly where sexuality is concerned. Recent studies of Puritanism have shown that the pervasive attitude toward sexuality was one of celebration of life's energies and its orders, such as marriage and love. While caricatures of Puritan attitudes have emphasized repression of natural bodily desires, a more accurate phrase for this mentality might be Weber's "worldly asceticism," a paradoxical attitude in which one loved this world without collapsing one's own moral standards. Hawthorne's portrayal of New England Puritan sexual attitudes in *The Scarlet Letter* captures a political, rather than a theological, world view. The town fathers (and the minister) use biblical phrases to serve political or personal ends, not simply judging Hester Prynne but tormenting her. Such hounding was, of course, inimical to the spirit of the New Testament, which elevated mercy over judgment and forgiveness over vengeance, where "in Christ we are set free" from the bondage of the law, and where Jesus released the woman taken in adultery, saying, "Go, and sin no more." The true Puritan ethos was fashioned not out of fear of impurity and degradation but in a more positive spirit of experiment, investigation, and imagination—in freedom, not in constriction.

That a healthy minded, life-centered attitude toward sexuality constituted the Reformed tradition's norm can be seen by examining the Westminster Confession, a document written by divines from various Calvinist parties. These representatives articulated the Reformed conception of marriage, love, and family life. "Marriage was ordained for the mutual help of husband and wife; for the increase of mankind with a legitimate issue, and of the church with an holy seal; and for preventing of uncleanness" (Westminster Confession, 24.2, p. 221). Marriage provides mutual aid and happiness; sustains the body, the human community, and the church; and directs sexual energies toward a fitting end. The Confession cautioned against consanguineous marriage, adultery, and fornication, drawing these warnings from the hygienic stipulations of the Levitical code of Israel. Further, these Calvinists laid great stress on the responsible selection of a mate ("a bonnie and brainie lassie"), attending to the Augustinian theme of corruption inhering in close or consanguineous unions and being aware of "hybrid vigor." Reproductive power and family covenant, the divines believed, provided an opportunity to bring into the world healthy, well-loved, and thoughtfully nurtured children. In the Calvinist view the natural processes were neither sacrosanct nor inevitable, as natural law had held, but involved choice and responsibility. Thus Reformed sex ethics emphasized the family covenant and the bond of love as these enriched the human community.

Marriage and family life were but one aspect of human sexuality. To an age in which sexual disturbance was often interpreted as witchcraft or

demoniac possession, the Puritan-reared Thomas Sydenham brought a human and liberating approach. In *Observationes Medicae* (1676) Sydenham,
one of the founders of clinical medicine, urged that we observe diseases in
and of themselves, rather than importing abstract theories (such as demoniac possession) to interpret the phenomena. "Nature by herself determines diseases," he wrote.[19] Sydenham's methods, combined with his humane approach to pathological disturbance, led to a less biased and more
sympathetic attitude toward sexual misbehavior. Most important, this
method enabled sexual and reproductive processes to be studied with an
objectivity and moral neutrality that allowed dispassionate, ultimately
helpful observations to be made. Sexuality is a powerful component in the
being of each of us, married or not.

Renaissance exuberance, with its exaltation of man's possibilities and its
celebration of human values, ultimately enriched our understanding of
sexuality. To the stimulation of sensible investigation, such as Sydenham's
in the seventeenth century, was added the perspective of eighteenth-
century Calvinist-influenced philosophers such as John Locke and David
Hume. This age of rational theology further developed the Reformation
themes of responsibility and conscience in family life, alongside a sense of
the beauty and joy of the natural world and the human body. Pleasure and
delight as aspects of sensation and reason were seen to be wholesome and
worthy of being celebrated.

For Friedrich Schleiermacher (and, earlier, for the American Calvinist
Jonathan Edwards), feelings were divine stirrings in the human spirit.
Schleiermacher wrote that human sexuality, conviviality, the birth of a
child, and the death of a friend are moments when our life in space and
time is touched by the infinite. At such grand moments of experience we
realize that "our own self is completely surrounded by the infinite," that
experiences "always stir a quiet longing and a holy reverence."[20] Fifteen
hundred years had elapsed since Augustine cautioned against passion.
Baptizing feelings—the human emotions of mercy, forgiveness, hope, sexual passion—with divine blessing countered the emergent mechanistic attitude toward the body that swept in with Descartes, Le Mettrie, and other
mathematical biologists. The clinical observations of Sydenham helped
clear the intellectual mists surrounding sexuality, but the obvious danger
of this scientific approach was to reduce human emotions to yet another
"function" in the workings of the "body-mind machine." Such dissection
would disjoin sexuality from its rightful place as the locus of the divine-
human encounter.

The romantic, liberal, and humanistic thrust of nineteenth-century Re-

formed theology, piety, and hymnody also challenged the reductionist tendency. Seizing on Luther's advice not to let the devil have all the good
tunes, the liturgy of the church began to associate the human love story
again with the divine drama of Christ's love for humankind. "I come to the
garden alone . . . I'll stay in the garden with Him. . . ." In these popular
love lyrics, which were later used as a prayer, human love was seen as con-
secrated by the Son of God, who crosses the vast cosmos in reconciling care
to find again his lost friend. The constant and faithful lover becomes the
prototype, the inspiration, indeed, the creator (God is love) of human trust
and fidelity.

In the nineteenth century F. D. Maurice sustained the biblical understanding of relationship that the Reformers had sought to articulate: that it
is anchored in, improved by, and guided by God. Love in this understanding is claimed for oneself but is also given away—it is amplified as it is extended. Love expressed within marriage diffuses itself through the house-
hold, "from the family it goes forth into the nation . . . where it is wanting,
society becomes an intolerable lie."[21] Maurice seems to believe that the entire social fabric coheres in this key relationship, the love between husband
and wife.

Barth, more than any other twentieth-century thinker, has articulated
the struggle of the Reformed tradition with the modern world. Liberated
by the sense of autonomy gained through the Enlightenment, secure in the
good life, yet horrified by the violence of our technological mass society,
we falter before the new choices thrust upon us in this new age. Choices no
longer center around marriage, or around the male-female relationship
generally, but now embrace all devices and activities concerned with the
consequences of the sexual encounter, such as birth control, childlessness,
and abortion.

All biomedical issues are dealt with by Barth in the context of an affir-
mative understanding of human sexuality. Barth's position is recognizably
biblical and Reformed: the male-female relationship is the locus of the
divine image. The sex relationship possesses "dignity" because it is the
"true creative image of God," a "type of the history of the covenant"
(*Dogmatics*, III/1). Relationship thus understood is no less than revolu-
tionary, for in this covenant woman (previously viewed as subordinate to
man in God's creation) is recognized as man's equal part in the *humanum*,
Adam. Such recognition of mutuality dignifies the relationship and the
shared common life of a couple.

Recent theological ethics tooled in the Reformed spirit have developed
two emphases in dealing with the wide spectrum of issues in human sex-

uality.[22] First, the primacy of the human, the relational, and the natural structures of existence determines the good; second, human liberation from the necessities of nature (genetics, childbearing, etc.) has been affirmed. The emancipation that God is bringing into our world not only releases us from death, transcience, and sin, but liberates us politically, economically, culturally, racially, and sexually, too.[23]

In struggling toward positions on the thorny issues of birth control, abortion, and the like, these thinkers (along with such others as Dietrich Ritschl and Jürgen Moltmann) have attempted to preserve a respect for human integrity and human needs.

Birth Control: For Barth the freedom of life fellowship is found in the intrinsic good of sexuality, a good not linked in the divine command to procreation. Its primary direction is the creation of marital fellowship. The act of generation and conception has its own intrinsic responsibility. Since the providence of God and "the course of nature" are not identical, the man/woman must affirm or deny in reason and will whether they are committing themselves to childbirth and its lifelong commitments. The blessing of God (a new child) demands the reciprocal *yes* of the man/woman (*Dogmatics*, III/4).

What are the implications of Reformed theology for conception-control and family planning? On the one hand, the husband and wife must decide together that pregnancy and childbirth can be endured, that the family has the strength to receive and nurture this new life; any signals that such an event would not be salutary (e.g., if the parents are carriers of a debilitating disease), would not honor God in his creation, should be taken seriously before pregnancy is sought. On the other hand, sometimes the grace of life is found not through deliberate reflection and planning but in surprise. Here the outstretched hand of God through the new creation should be thankfully celebrated. A couple should, in other words, combine the attitudes of responsibility and receptivity.

Childlessness: The new technological capacities for insemination and conception have raised moral questions about the problems of childlessness: seeking one's own biological offspring through the techniques of artificial insemination, in vitro fertilization, or surrogate motherhood. In general, the Reformed tradition would not endorse the desire of modern couples to remain childless unless there were very strong reasons, such as the survival and health of the marriage or the sensed vocation and life purpose experienced by this man and woman before God. While the modern arguments of career advancement and economic inadequacy are compelling and understandable, they do not seem to justify this no to God and human history in refusing the gift of life.

The desire to have one's own genetic offspring although one or both partners are sterile presents a more difficult problem. The passion to generate new life from one's own being is commendable within the ethical tradition of the church. But bitterness over one's own debility and a demand to create offspring "like us" when so many parentless children remain unclaimed seems a questionable attitude. The emotional, physical, and economic costs of in vitro fertilization and surrogate motherhood are so great that one must ask whether such desire to parent a child constitutes gracious acceptance of new life or a demand for biological immortality.

The complex of desires, emotions, and ambitions of which we speak is illustrated by the case of a Midwestern woman who agreed to carry the artificially inseminated offspring of a New York man. When the child was born deformed by microcephaly, the gentleman refused to pay the ten-thousand-dollar fee to the mother. For a brief and painful time no one wanted the poor baby. The case was formally settled when the woman and her husband accepted the child as their own after tests had shown the baby to have been fathered by the woman's husband. The new sexual technologies will create chaos if they are not used with responsibility and care.

Case Study: Abortion

The Reformed tradition has also pondered the difficult question of abortion. Presbyterian policy has emphasized two values: the respect for life and the personal conscience and choice of parents. Barth has argued that the grace of freedom in life together bears the command of God to respect and protect persons. We are also invited, not coerced, to freely decide for God and the good. But Christian freedom in the biblical-Augustinian-Reformed tradition is not autonomy. Confusing the Reformation doctrine of conscience with the Enlightenment notion of autonomy has been misleading. Christian freedom is receptivity to the divine Word to honor life in each other. Human existence is by its very nature covenant partnership with God, which means being for and with others (*Mitmenschlichkeit*). God's nature determines human nature as convivial, given in concern to one another.

From relatedness to the other flow the imperatives of respect and protection of life. God is for us and for all peoples. He wills life, extends the grace of life in the miracle of conception. He alone has authority to end life. But even life itself is not the *summum bonum*. This belongs only to the commanding God. Barth has an intriguing passage relating the sovereignty of the Word to human freedom:

> Human life, and therefore the life of the unborn child, is not an absolute, so that, while it can be protected by the commandment, it can be so only within the limits of the will of Him who issues it.... In His grace God can will to preserve the life which He has given, and in His grace He can will to take it again. Either way it is not lost before Him. Men cannot exercise the same sovereignty in relation to it. It does not really lie in their power even to preserve it.... Let us be quite frank and say that there are situations in which the killing of germinating life does not constitute murder but is in fact commanded. (*Dogmatics*, III/4, pp. 420–21)

This passage is crucial to any formulation of a Reformed ethics of abortion. At one level it contends that only God has the authority (power) to give or take life and, therefore, only a misuse of human power can cause one person to take the life of another. A modern philosopher makes the same point:

> Perhaps the most fundamental moral intuition is that it is wrong to take the life of another human being. Nearly as fundamental, however, is the intuition that under certain circumstances it is permissible to do so.[24]

This passage from Baruch Brody's study *Abortion and the Sanctity of Human Life* resonates with the convictions that appear in the sensitized Christian conscience as it ponders the issue of abortion. When we are close to Christ and responsive to his will in our thinking and acting, the primary value that is born in our spirit is that life is infinitely precious and should not be violated. However, this primary value is followed by another value that allows for the existence of particular and exceptional circumstances when we face the tragic necessity of bringing a human life, our own or that of another, to its end.

Abortion is a "borderline situation," an *ultima ratio*. Since the command of God and the will of Christ weighs against it, it cannot be undertaken unless all alternatives have been exhausted. But if or when it becomes the last recourse, then in the crisis of that decision it may become the command of God under the release of his grace. The posture of the Christian community is not to condemn, but to stand by with forgiveness and support.

This point devolves on the essential genius of the Christian Gospel ethic as conveyed to us in the Reformed tradition. God is for us. His will for us is freedom to be his friends, to be partners with others in the liberating human quest, to be builders and redeemers. His Word is our joy, our life. In the service of Christ we are released to the creative freedom and power of his will. In the context of faith, any act cannot be right or wrong in itself. It is either compatible or incompatible within the relationship with Christ. The commandment of God, the living and written word, the immediacy of divine command within the conscience, instruct us as we search for appropriate moral responses within this relation. Barth confided: "There will be situations in which all those concerned must answer before God in great loneliness and secrecy, and make their decision accordingly" (*Dogmatics*, III/4, p. 421).

Three themes of Calvinistic social ethics seem particularly relevant to the abortion question: toleration, prudence, and conscience. In the seventeenth century, physician-philosopher John Locke, the son of a Puritan justice, formulated the doctrine of religious and political toleration. This principle, appropriated by Jefferson, Madison, and other American political philosophers, guided the formation of our governmental system. Reformed ethics has always sought a political philosophy built on respect for diverse positions on questions of belief and morals. Presbyterian cultures in Bohemia, France, Switzerland, Scotland, and America have exemplified this principle.

John Locke, like the seventeenth-century Puritans, believed in two sources of morality. First, there was the positive law of the will of God. This revealed law was known in Scripture and in conscience. The other source of morality was human reason. To common sense and prudence the laws of nature were self-evident: as in mathematics, there was a logical development from basic principles to middle axioms to specific stipulates for action. In Locke's system the commands of God and common sense coalesced into a structure of law that would guide public life. Government, however, was not to intervene where the law of God was silent. In areas of the legal social contract, popular law had force. In all other areas people should enjoy freedom. The least government is the best government, according to Locke. The underlying theological premise of this scheme was Calvin's unique blending of Roman law, the Bible, Augustine, and Luther, which had three points: first, the absolute sovereignty of God and his will within the personal conscience; second, the recognition of the propensity of will to power and exploitation among people, especially in their relations with each other, and, third, that therefore the basis of the social contract should be a strong allegiance to the state, which ought to exercise limited power. Humans exist, according to Locke, to live for God's glory in worship and to maintain a just and benevolent society.[25]

The doctrine of religious and moral toleration was formed, under Presbyterian and Puritan influence, by the Scottish and French philosophers, Milton's debate with Hobbes, and Locke's own reflections, under the influence of his mentor and patron Lord Shaftesbury. Locke's position hinged on his doctrine of "indifference." Some issues, he felt, clearly mandated in faith, belonged in the church and, therefore, should not be interfered with by the state. Other powers resided in the state, and here the church or private opinion should have no influence. Issues in the moral sphere, especially issues of human sexuality, such as abortion, belonged in the realm of "indifferent" items, and prudence required that they be regulated by neither church nor state.

In the Reformed tradition the third vector of ethics is conscience. As human beings, created *imago dei*, we are imbued with two senses that perceive God and moral truth. The *sensus divinitatis* is the direct awareness of God in the human soul as mediated through nature and reason. *Consciencia* is the subjective revelation of God and his will to the personal soul. As Calvin has written:

> There are two principal parts of the light which still remains in corrupt nature: first, the seed of religion is implanted in all men; next, the distinction between good and evil is engraved in their consciences.[26]

Here Calvin was referring explicitly to the Greek *prolapses*, the faculty for discerning the requirements of rectitude and justice. Conscience is a "knowing with," an interactive phenomenon. It is a knowledge formed in the relationship of the person to God within the polarity of good and evil.[27] Conscience is the vehicle by which God communicates his good will and his judgment to the individual. This doctrine admits none of the cultural relativity of the anthropological understanding of conscience or the psychodynamic interpretations of the Freudian model.

This most persuasive motif in Calvin's theology bears "the terrible choice" of abortion. Several elements become clear: first, that choice belongs in the inner citadel of a person's (or a family's) relationship with God; second, that the dialectics of judgment and grace frame the decision (this is especially true when profound goods and evils inhere in a single decision); third, that the decision and subsequent support (either gracious forgiveness or generous cooperation and undergirding) belong within the faith community. When the individuals involved are separated from this fellowship, the caring community must reach out in Christ's spirit with ministries of counseling, mutual aid, and care for unwed mothers.

In collective conscience the church should expend its witness in prophetic and pastoral influences rather than through political control. The church should hold forth a vision of personal and societal righteousness and the requirement of social justice. In the area of sexuality and procreation this prophetic stance will condemn the pornographic and the licentious fascination of our culture, with its degrading portrayal of the lurid, the base, and the promiscuous. Rather, it will proffer the vision of loving and respectful human relations, responsible sexuality, and vibrant and caring family life. The prophetic command will call society to its obligation of mutual care and service. Pastorally, the church should go to the dark and desperate places where brokenness, alienation, sin, and suffering are found and there extend the mercy and life-remoralizing power of Christ. A new quality of sexual chastity and personal responsibility often follows when, in Christ's name, someone cares.

In the Reformed tradition both moral and public policy will be grounded in a mingling of the imperatives gained by toleration, reason, and conscience. Abortion is homicide. The subtleties of reasoning that seek to establish subhumanness or subpersonhood in the fetus simply do not work. Abortion presents a tough conflict between the interests of persons that must be arbitrated in a vigorous way. The ancient Jewish notion of a fetus being in some cases an unjust aggressor, making an unacceptable claim on a woman's life-support system, has some credence. Abortion is in some situations justifiable homicide.

This ethical analysis should require that we morally differentiate abortion cases along a spectrum. It is simplistic to say that abortion is always right or always wrong. Even though philosophy demands consistency and the law requires uniformity, other criteria should be applied when making decisions involving persons' lives. We need, therefore, to distinguish among differing situations and admit that there are times when the technique of abortion must be used. In the public-policy arena we need to develop an ethic of reason and prudence. Then, in a nuanced way, we can assign value or disvalue to a given case according to some balance of the principles of beneficence, nonmaleficence, justice, and freedom. A suggestive grouping of cases might be these: abortion is *strongly advised* in cases of incest and child rape, where profound genetic defect is present, or in life-threatening pregnancy, for example. Abortion is *permissible but not obligatory* in cases of out-of-wedlock pregnancy, where pregnancy presents a physical or mental risk to the mother, and when moderately severe genetic or congenital abnormalities are discovered in the fetus. Abortion is *permissible but discouraged* in illegitimate pregnancies, and in cases of mild and treatable genetic or congenital accidents. Abortion is *strongly discouraged* for sex-selection or population control.

Abortion is a crisis for each of us, but for a particular group it is a prevalent dilemma. This group is young (fifteen to twenty-five years old), unmarried women who become pregnant. In 1978, 75 percent of those who sought abortions in the United States were unmarried. Thirty percent of the total 1.4 million were under twenty years of age, and 65 percent were under twenty-five. In other words, nearly one million abortions were performed in 1978 for young, unmarried women. The principal moral phenomenon we are dealing with, therefore, is that of a great proportion (perhaps 10 percent) of our young-adult female population finding themselves in an unacceptable trap from which they seek release. These women are not proud or particularly guilty, they simply find themselves in trouble and need help. Before condemning or exhorting these women, the church must extend mercy. Emulating Christ, who drew near to the lost and the broken, the church should be in the trenches with those who suffer, rather than standing aloof in contempt and righteous indignation. The pilgrimage of grace is a story of repentance, restitution, and regeneration. The mercy of God and the grace of Christ go out to the extreme boundaries of our evil and estrangement. The church must abide in and offer that grace.

·4·

Acting Human:
Life's Choices and Destiny

MORALITY

Christian ethics . . . is the reflection upon the question, and its answer: What
am I, as a believer in Jesus Christ and as a member of his church, to do?[1]

The personality develops, or it withers, as it passes along its life course.
How does a person who is and is becoming make moral choices? Does he
act within the context of faith-communal ethics (*koinōnia*) or does he act
autonomously? This section on morality relies considerably on the work of
a major Presbyterian ethicist and theologian, Paul Lehmann. Lehmann's
discussion of *koinōnia* ethics, the ethics of a biblically covenanted people,
in Israel and the primitive church, in classic Christian and Reformation
perspective, best presents both the particularity and the universality of the
Calvinist tradition.

The crux of ethics theologically conceived is sensitivity to, and movement along with, the ruling, reconciling, and redeeming activity of God in
the world. The ancients spoke of ethics as knowing and doing the will of
God. For Lehmann, the Reformed tradition introduced a liberating grasp
of the ways of God with men and thus also the possibility of ever fresh and
experimental responses to the dynamics and the humanizing character of
the divine activity in the world (p. 14). Ethics is the bringing of our personal
and collective willing and deciding to coincide with what "God is doing in
the world to make and keep human life human," Lehmann continues.
Aware of our propensity to want to undo what God has done (natural law)
and what he is doing (redemptive purpose), we need constantly to be reclaimed to theonomy, God's moral purpose. In Calvin and the Puritan tradition, piety is the creative force stimulating that conformation. Remembering the Sabbath—indeed, keeping holy the divine plantation in our times,

places, and lives (which includes conscience)—is the secret of the coadventure with God. Jeremy Taylor's great confessions, *Holy Living and Holy Dying*,[2] witnessed to exactly this inextricable interdependence of piety and ethics.

When it comes to designating "what God is doing in the world" or what activity constitutes the divine rule, we immediately confront the Reformation principle, so strong in Calvin and Barth, that God is wholly other, not available to our control, inscrutable in his purposes, and obscure (*deus absconditas*) in his being. One risks pretense and pride when one claims to have identified "what God is doing in the world." But we are driven back to revelation. The story of God's dealing with Israel, the Gospel statement of the career of Jesus, the apostolic activity (preaching, healing, baptizing, remembering the eucharist) in which the Christ event becomes for us the continuation of God's covenant with Israel, all portray to us what God is doing in the world, in history, with real people. Ongoing history is now the continuation of the divine story (*Heilsgeschichte*), since creation, incarnation, and sanctification (that is, the Holy Spirit making the world new) assure the ongoing narrative. God has made the history of planet Earth his story. To see what God is doing in the world, wrote Karl Barth, we read with the Bible in one hand and the newspaper in the other.[3]

Our problem is not that of knowing what God is doing or what his will is—our problem is doing it: going along in his way. The existence and activity of God are self-evident to reason, as Paul said:

> All that may be known of God by men lies plainly before their eyes; indeed God himself has disclosed it to them. His invisible attributes, that is to say his everlasting power and deity, have been visible, ever since the world began, to the eye of reason, in the things he has made . . . yet knowing God they have refused to honor him as God. (Rom. 1:19–20)

The law of God is restated in various versions: detailed (613 commandments), abbreviated (ten words) or simplified (What does the Lord require of you but to do justice, "love mercy and walk humbly with your God"? "Love the Lord your God with all your heart, with all your soul, with all your mind and with all your strength. . . . Love your neighbor as yourself." —Mic. 6:6–8; Mark 12:29–31; Deut. 6:5; Lev. 19:18).

The divine being and activity are self-evident and universal to moral reason, to Kant as to Paul in Romans, through "the starry heavens above and the moral law within." Yet Kant, like the young Augustine (before he was coerced into ordination), was not impressed with the Old Testament story as an expression of God's nature and activity. God's pure being and will was one thing, but the messy and offensive story of the patriarchs was another.

In the Bible story we are confronted with "Israel's life-and-death passion for transmitting a tradition" (Buber). This tradition, incorporated at every stage of composition and canonization, has two motifs: God's persistent care and rule and our persistent resistance and will to power. God delivers, the people forget. God provides a home, the people construe it as their accomplishment. God creates a theocracy, the people demand monarchy. God smashes, scatters, and reestablishes, the people take power into their own hands. The Messiah institutes his reign, the people insist on their own devices and rituals: "We have a law and by that law he must die" (John 19:7).

All along the way Israel's friendship with God has been affirmed by following and denied by departing from God's way. Moral rectitude seals the relationship. The moral purpose given as the human side of the covenant arrangement is what God is doing in the world. He is liberating the oppressed. He is feeding the hungry. He is bringing justice to communities and nations. He is creating love as the binding fabric of life in this world. God creates the conditions for human fulfillment. He commands what he wills and gives what he commands. His purposes for the world can be brought about only by the life and actions of his people.

When we turn, then, to the narrow spectrum of issues surrounding human birth, life, death, sexuality, suffering, and the like, we see certain clear values that indicate moral imperatives: the survival of the lives that God has given, the enhancement of those lives, and the generation of a continuing human family. Morality has thus a singularly positive function. Destructive action is allowed only for the containment of power that would destroy those values.

As we discuss more specifically "what God is doing in the world," we discover the complexity and difficulty of ethics. The broad directions of the divinely given good life are clear. The necessity for pure and active association (piety) with God in order to know and will the good is implied. The formation of personal character that instinctively recognizes and responds to moral imperatives is also desirable. The requirement to resist even to the point of suffering those malign forces in life is likewise a divine given. The difficulty comes as the ethical requirement makes greater and greater demands on us, for neither righteous statements nor correct overt action suffice. Our sentiments, dispositions, and wills must be given over to God and his good will. The rich young man who confronted Jesus asked:

'Master, what good must I do to gain eternal life?' 'Good?' responded Jesus, 'Why do you ask me about that? One alone is good. But if you wish to enter into life, keep the commandments.' 'Which commandments?' he asked. Jesus answered, 'Do not murder; do not commit adultery; do not steal, do not give false evidence; honor your father and mother; and love your neighbor as yourself.' The young man answered, 'I have kept all these. Where do I still fall short?' Jesus said to him, 'If you wish to go the whole way, go sell all your possessions, and give to the poor, and then you will have riches in heaven; and come, follow me.' When the young man heard this, he went away with a heavy heart; for he was a man of great wealth. (Matt. 19: 16–22)

The story of the rich young ruler shows that morality entails not merely keeping the commandments (that is, leading what would be called commonly the "good" or "virtuous" life) but surrendering the total self—goods, will, life—to Christ.

Ethics, then, like health, sexuality, and passages, is a matter of abandonment, of giving way to God and the other. Ethics involves not valuing any penultimate thing. Ethics, which comes from God, rather than being a human artifact, is following in a way that may, indeed, will, demand that everything else be put aside. When we face issues of genetic manipulation, modification of human sexual and procreative activity, fundamental controls over human mentality and behavior, even control over the process of dying, we see the helpful guidance of the specific commands (vitality, chastity, honesty, integrity, charity). We also see the necessity of those deeper pillars of moral commitment that undergird overt behaviors. What we will to do and choose to do must be given to God and be excellent for our fellow men. All hidden ulterior motives must be cleansed; otherwise the most upright actions can be destructive. Ethics involves character and volition, as well as thought and act.

Today we find ourselves in a social setting that the Bible writers could not have anticipated. We are no longer merely the passive receivers of life, innocent participants in the world of association with fellow humanity and the natural world. We have been given in the providence of God the power of self-creation and a profound control over the quality and dynamic of our own existence. The environment is plastic to our will, even to the point of collapse. The opportunity to follow divine guidance is a blessed grace in this frightening age. It is in exhilarating freedom that we enjoy being able to contour our creative thought and technique to a divine purpose. At the same time the temptation to frustrate, rather than follow, will be strong. The arrogance of power in self-serving and exploitation will continue to tempt us.

Ethics as "Koinōnia" or Autonomy

The genius of Christian ethics is not only its grounding in the divine purpose but its setting in a communal tradition. Lehmann exposits Reformed ethics as *koinōnia* ethics, the ethics of a called and covenanted community, a people with a peculiar destiny—to spearhead God's working in the world. This community, called *ekklēsia* ("those set apart in the way"), is the Hebrew congregation and the Christian fellowship. The people of God are the people of the way, the people who follow Moses' God, "who is becoming who he will be" (Exod. 3:14). This people is the people of "the age to come." The reality that animates life and action in this community is proleptic and prophetic. It anticipates what God is bringing, and acts to bring it about. This people also lives out a prophetic existence by instrumentally allowing God to usher his intended creation into the world that is coming to be. Prophecy is fore-telling and forth-telling what is in favor of what ought to be and will soon be.

The people of "the age to come" are a saving community who bring life and health to the dying and sick. They move out to the perimeters of the world, the abandoned regions victimized by the exploitative power of the mighty. They bring the message of liberation and salvation. Through the Holy Spirit, which in ethics is the continual pointer to the will and power of Christ (John 16:12–15), the community lives not unto itself, but unto him who calls it into being. The essence of *koinōnia* ethics is given in Paul's letter to a cell of that body in Ephesus.

> To me, though I am the very least of all the saints, this grace was given, to preach to the gentiles the unsearchable riches of Christ, and to make all men see what is the plan of the mystery hidden for ages in God who created all things; that through the church [*dia tās ecclesias*] the manifold wisdom of God might now be made known to the principalities and powers in the heavenly places. This was according to the eternal purpose which he has realized in Christ Jesus our Lord, in whom we have boldness and confidence of access through our faith in him. . . .
>
> For this reason I bow my knees before the Father, . . . that according to the riches of his glory he may grant you to be strengthened with might through his Spirit in the inner man, and that Christ may dwell in your hearts through faith; that you, being rooted and grounded in love, may have power to comprehend with all the saints what is the breadth and length and height and depth, and to know the love of Christ which surpasses knowledge, that you may be filled with all the fullness of God. . . .
>
> I, therefore, a prisoner for the Lord, beg you to lead a life worthy of the

calling to which you have been called, with all lowliness and meekness, with patience, forbearing one another in love, eager to maintain the unity of the Spirit in the bond of peace. (Eph. 3:8–4:3)

Koinōnia ethics is at once theonomous and heteronomous. It is autonomous only in the sense that it allows no other institution or power to rule morally in the soul. Moral direction is conviction in the soul responding to divine command and human justice. What we are to be and do is given us by God through the community with others: the believing fellowship and the larger human community. We are not autonomous (self-ruling) creatures. We belong to and live for one another because our Father has joined us into one body, one family. Directions for personal action are indicated by that which is needed to edify the community. My desire may be for self-aggrandizement and self-glorification, but the pressure of my call, my "vocation" (Calvin), and my membership in *ekklēsia* and *koinōnia* lay on me another claim. My gifts—not developed powers, but divine gifts—have been given for service to the world. They must be expressed for the whole story to proceed, the whole architecture to continue.

The alternative to theocentric and altruistic ethics is the ethics of autonomy. During the nineteenth century the human agent was declared free from the tyranny of ecclesial, political, and psychological hegemony. The movement of modern times has been in the direction of free and unbridled self-rule. While the Christian ethic indeed sets one free, it is not the absolute freedom of the Enlightenment but freedom in responsibility. Philosophical ethics are man-made ethics. In this view the moral task is neither adhering to an undergirding natural law nor perceiving and obeying a divine command; rather, ethics constructs the most sensible and reasonable way to live and act. Joseph Fletcher, who has moved from theological to autonomous ethics in his own thought, argues that God, if such exists, would surely concur with the postulates of mutual respect and agape love that are the noblest expressions of our moral reason.[4]

Autonomous ethics is also formulated over against the ethics of paternalism. Building on John Stuart Mill's discussion *On Liberty*, which argues that individuals should be able to choose their own actions unless those actions threaten harm to others, scholars such as Gerald Dworkin contend that the society should regulate behavior only when it shows sufficient danger in nonregulation and when the governed freely consent.[5]

At one level, the insistence on human autonomy in ethics lies very much in the spirit of the Jewish and Christian understanding of persons as free and dignified agents who owe allegiance only to God and their personal conscience. At another level, however, we have here a utilitarian and Enlightenment image of the person as a detached island with no binding connections to any other. *Koinōnia* ethics, in contrast, acknowledges that we exist for one another and not for ourselves—as in the case of the father who ordered his son to submit to a blood test requested for a study on a blood disorder not affecting the boy himself. Against the boy's initial refusal (saying it was "his body") stands the spirit of the biblical tradition, wherein our own freedoms and comforts are sometimes subordinated to our sense of solidarity with the human family.

The other serious problem that Reformed ethics finds with the autonomy tradition is the underlying assumption that man is a self-determining creature. Apart from any contention that self-determination works or doesn't work according to some utilitarian calculus, biblical ethics rejects the assumption of man's self-determination. Because of the divine election, wrote Barth, "the question arises concerning the self-determination of man in the light of his determination by God" (*Dogmatics*, II/2, p. 575). Autonomy ethics capitulates to the egoistic flaw in human nature, where all good is seen as revolving around one's own needs and wants. Ethics in this spirit is not motivated by deep sympathy for fellow humans but by self-assertion and advocacy of rights. The style of human interactions founded on this underlying anthropology is the modern state, where individuals, defended by their lawyers, are constantly asserting and defending their "rights." Morally speaking, this development represents only a slight advance from that state described by Machiavelli, in which power and influence defined justice.

Ethics in the Reformed Tradition

When we turn to older moral traditions that live on today in the Reformed branch of the Christian family, we find that certain tendencies and positions have recurred. In primitive moral awareness, that which offended God also presumably destroyed humans. Such offenses against God were restrained by making certain zones of experience sacrosanct. Offenses against other persons and the natural world (which is spirited) were prohibited by taboos.

To stand for truth and good was to stand with and for God. For Socrates, and within the profound moral consciousness that developed around the Mediterranean basin (Egypt, Western Asia, Greece), love of God meant moral purity. Moral impurity was synonymous with idolatry. Plato wrote in the *Theaetetus*:

> In the divine there is no shadow of unrighteousness, only the perfection of righteousness. Nothing is more like the divine than any one of us who becomes as righteous as possible. It is here that a man shows his true spirit and power or lack of spirit and nothingness. For to know this is wisdom and excellence of the genuine sort; not to know it is to be manifestly blind and base.[6]

It is the righteousness of God manifesting itself in human actions and decisions that renders a person righteous, moral, or truly human. To the Hebrews, being bound to God in faith involved being bound to fellow humanity in holy covenant. Obligations ensued between fathers and children, children and elders, husbands and wives, clansmen and strangers. These obligations were detailed both in positive demands (respect, mercy, forgiveness, justice) and in negative restraints (do not kill, steal, tempt, deceive). All these specific ethical requirements radiated from a core notion of what faithful relations demanded because these relations were bestowed within the covenant of divine fidelity with us. For the Jew, righteousness conveyed health, fertility, longevity, and peace. Disobedience brought shame, disease, and, if not death, sadness and vexation. For this reason God's people called by his name "delight in his law."

Jews and Christians are communities of moral law. Law, in its wholesome sense, is not restrictive constraint but liberating power to realize and sustain humanness. Law is the substance of the divine expectation. Obedience is our answer to God about what makes for health and salvation. The Jewish tradition remains a tradition of law. Talmud, Mishna, and medical *halacha* build on the fundaments of Torah. The relation of underlying righteousness and basic principles to specific cases is articulated in the counsel of rabbis down through the ages. Precedent builds on previous wisdom. The Roman Catholic casuistic tradition and Protestant case ethics build upon this Hebraic foundation.

A central theme of the New Testament is that Christ has achieved what the law could not. He is the righteousness of God, righteousness which might be defined as "liberating justice." Jesus Christ is the decisive act of God to make right what had gone wrong. Righteousness is now made manifest through Christ. The profound center of ethical teaching in the New Testament is Paul's Letter to the Romans. In this, the most magnificent and searching theological argument ever presented, Paul claims that Christ has confronted us not only with the perfect moral demand but with the fulfillment of that demand. Jesus has reminded us of the rigor of the ethical requirement. Outward righteousness must be undergirded by a heart surrendered to God alone. Hebrew ethics—total love of God, and love for neighbor measured by self-love—were deep and searching. The facile legalism of the technicians of law missed the mark. Even the impressive piety of the Pharisees did not go to the heart. It went far—that is why Jesus dealt so seriously with it—but it came up short. Ethics was a matter of act, mind, will, and heart, all in the service of the objective good, God's will.

Paul's rendition of ethics released both moral truth and a dangerous disorder into Christian history. If Christ fulfills all righteousness, related-ness to him and strenuous coparticipation in his new creation constitutes the very essence of morality. This same strength can be used as a moral escape, however. Paul, who had personally known the disorienting effect of Jewish works-righteousness, was overwhelmed by the justifying grace of God in Christ. In his enthusiasm he concentrated attention on Christian liberty and freedom from the law. This revolution in ethical insight be-stowed the grace of emancipated, Christocentric conscience on all who would receive Jesus as Lord. This would become the essential feature of ethics in the Reformed tradition. It remained to the *koinōnia* context of Pauline teaching, the penetration of Stoic casuistry, and the continuing Jewish-Christian doctrine of James and Jerusalem Christianity to retain substantive content within early Christian ethics. These three augmenta-tions saved the ethics of the early church from antinomianism, the fore-runner of autonomy ethics.

Initially, Paul was confronted by a dizzy spectrum of practices in the new churches, especially those in Greece and Asia Minor. This variety of sexual, ritual, and liturgical expressions, founded on the liberating spirit of the Gospel and Paul's interpretation of it, dismayed those who craved order and uniformity. This dazzling freedom also led some to the brink of crip-pling licentiousness and created confusion among the young converts. To this threat Paul brought the simple counsel: "all things are lawful but not all things are helpful ["expedient"]" (1 Cor. 6:12). A simple test added to the sense of freedom in conscience was the question of whether actions helped people along in their nascent life in Christ or offended and caused stumbling. *Koinōnia* ethics served the body, the building; it was edifying.

From Judaism and Hellenism, early Christian ethics retained the lists of common duties. Rudolf Bultmann has shown how the *Haustafeln* (house-hold duties) were absorbed into Christian morality from Hellenistic Judaism and Stoicism.[7] These lists of virtues and vices were baptized into Christian service, but here they took on a completely new reference. These habits flowed from the axis of a redeemed human heart living no longer to law (particularly not to moral dicta) or flesh, but to the spirit in Christ. As the apocalyptic fervor wore off and the church settled back into history, instruction developed as a careful guidance into good and holy living that would become the ethical code, the "situation ethics," for subsequent Christian generations. The emerging table followed the prescriptive and proscriptive style of the Noachian and Covenant codes:

Virtues	Vices	
love	stealing	quarrelsomeness
joy	injustice	contentiousness
peace	fornication	ambition
patience	idolatry	dissension
kindness	adultery	intrigue
goodness	homosexuality	jealousy
fidelity	drunkenness	mischief
gentleness	slander	rapacity
self-control	swindling	malice
loyalty to parents	impurity	murder
conscientiousness	indecency	insolence
	sorcery	arrogance
	envy	deceitfulness
	rage	

(Matt. 5:3–12, 25–26, 31–32; Gal. 5:19–23; 1 Cor. 5:10–11, 6:9–10; 2 Cor. 6:14–7:1; Rom. 1:28–32, 13:13; Col. 2:20–3:17; Rev. 21:8, 22:14–15)

Again, the human moral agent, rather than being imprisoned by the "nots," was released by the "shalts": The whole of the law may be summarized thusly: "Love the Lord your God with all your heart . . . and your neighbor as yourself."

Moreover, the prophetic Jewish ethic influenced early Christian attitudes toward morality. The work of James and the Jerusalem Christian community echoed the themes of high Judaism: justice to the poor, correspondence of word and deed, and strong insistence that faith necessarily issues in works. These three moral ideas, along with the specific instruction of the Gospels, the imitation of Christ legacy, and the specific Pauline moral instruction, formed the New Testament ethic. This entire superstructure was built on the new insight of Christ as the righteousness of God and forgiver of human sin.

One further element that influenced New Testament ethical teachings must be mentioned. A sense of impending judgment has receded from modern ethical consciousness, but early Christians lived under the ominous and liberating specter of final judgment. In the stark imagery of Jude, evil persons are

> clouds carried away by the wind without
> Giving rain, trees that in season bear no fruit,
> Dead twice over and pulled up by the roots.
> They are fierce waves of the sea, foaming
> Shameful deeds; they are stars that have
> Wandered from their course.
> And the place forever reserved for them is blackest darkness.
> (Jude 12–13)

We are to be moral—first, because of God's nature and, second, because righteousness heals and fulfills our own nature, while vice harms and destroys. But third, as this passage implies, vindication awaits the good, and condemnation the evil, person, now and at death. The people who built the medieval cathedrals and those who knew Dante and Milton by heart or were moved by the paintings of Masaccio and Michelangelo or the music of Bach knew vividly the moral demand. The tympanums at Vézelay and Autun represent a scenario that the medieval, like the early Christian, mind could not forget: that at the Last Judgment the Lord would appear in his majesty and all our deeds would be laid bare, weighed on the scale of justice.

Such fear of judgment and anticipation of reward has had an ambivalent effect on the history of ethics. While the belief that one day each must give account for his life (from the Egyptian concept of weighing Tut's heart on the scales of justice to the hell-fire preaching of the Puritans) often served to guide and motivate ethical behavior in a salutary way, often, too, this idea demeaned the free and spontaneous will that God implanted in our conscience. It coerced *orthopraxis* (good deeds) without *orthodoxa* (good heart). Early Christian ethics firmly planted in the human soul the notion that humans are moral beings, responsible and accountable. Such an idea inhered in the awareness that God is moral and purposive and that therefore the human personality is of infinite value.

A consideration of the moral life preoccupied Augustine as much as it had his predecessors. God, wrote Augustine, was *fons justitiae, sol justitiae, summa justitiae* (*C.D.* 1.21, 5.16, 20.2). Concentration on this Pauline vision of God in Christ as both the source and the fulfillment of righteousness led Augustine into the unfortunate position of advocating two moralities: a higher calling with a more searching demand, and the layman's ethic. Apart from this disorientation, which has so often appeared in religious history, Augustine's system constitutes the majestic groundwork for all subsequent reflection on ethics.

According to Augustine, God is both the moral demand and the moral resource (against the Pelagian emphasis on man as formulator of moral goals and source of moral power). The heathen virtues are "splendid vices" in that they serve human life nobly when sanctified by the grace of Christ. Platonic ideals, Stoic soul disciplines, and Epicurean affections all serve to harmonize order and beautify our life when God is acknowledged as the source of good. Ideals and rules are important in ethics. Augustine could never forsake the moral genius of Plato and Cicero: everything in its place and in pursuit of its inherent purpose is ethical fulfillment. "The body's peace. . . . is an orderly disposition of the parts thereof . . . a reasonable soul's. . . . a true harmony between knowledge and performance" (*C.D.* 9.13). Reason and rhetoric, thought and deliberation, are windows for seeing and doing the good.

Calvin, the lawyer-theologian, was deeply steeped in Seneca's ethic and in teleological natural law as mediated through the Augustinian-Thomist tradition. Since good proceeds from God, ethics confirms salvation. Good work and obedience to the divine law do not merit salvation but are rather symptomatic evidence of underlying righteousness. Calvinism, in contrast with Luther's ethic, laid great stress on good works as evidence of salvation.

The debate between Thomas More and William Tyndale in the early 1530s illustrated the ethical direction the Calvinist ethical tradition followed at the time of the Reformation. Medieval Catholic casuistry had taken the Augustinian celebration of classic virtues and formed it into a canonical system of moral truth. In Thomas Aquinas the rational structure of morality lived alongside revealed moral truth as a single standard. This system, blending elements drawn from archaic and Hebrew morality, from classic Greek and Roman philosophy and law, and from the church fathers, became normative to ethics as Thomism became normative for doctrine. When the medieval synthesis began to break down, the early Protestants (Wycliffe, Hus, Waldo, and, eventually, Luther and Calvin) were accused of antinomianism. Since they believed God alone (not the church tradition or the pope) was lord of the conscience, and that Scripture alone was authoritative in faith and morals, they could not accept the Thomist system of ethics.

Thomas More, the great apologist for the inherited substance of Catholic moral teaching, apparently had accused Tyndale, a Reformer, of lawlessness. Tyndale replied in a series of essays that the Reformed stream of Catholic ethics was not antinomian; rather, it situated the law in a very central place. But the new accent was not on the power of the law to make one right but on moral living as evidence of underlying salvation.

> All the good promises which are made us throughout all the Scripture . . . are all made us on this condition and covenant on our party, that we henceforth love the law of God, to walk therein, and to do it, and fashion our lives thereafter . . . there is no promises made him, but to them only that promise to keep the law.[8]

Tyndale said that true faith, as opposed to false faith, issues in love for God's law.

Tyndale maintained that lawful living is conditionally linked to salvation: "None of us can be received to grace but upon a condition to keep the law."[9] 2 Peter 1:10 became the watchword of Calvinists and Puritans. Indeed, it became the essence of the Presbyterian ethos: "Exert yourselves to clinch God's choice of calling you." All the Reformed catechisms of the sixteenth and seventeenth centuries reflected this concentration on moral law. Extensive commentary on the Ten Commandments can be found in the Heidelberg and French Calvinist catechisms, the Scots Confession of 1560, the Swiss documents, and the Westminster Catechism of 1646. A "good conscience" became the primary evidence of saving faith for Calvinists in England, Holland, and New England.

Indeed, a good conscience became the motivation to do more good works. God in Christ was seen as the provider of, and stimulus to, ethical actions:

> The cause of good works, we confess, is not our free will, but the spirit of the Lord Jesus, who dwells in our hearts by true faith, brings forth such works as God has prepared for us to walk in. (Scots Confession, ch. 13, p. 67)

> Good works, done in obedience to God's commandments, are the fruits and evidences of a true and lively faith; and by them believers manifest their thankfulness, strengthen their assurance, edify their brethren, adorn the profession of the Gospel, stop the mouths of adversaries, and glorify God whose workmanship they are, created in Christ Jesus therefore unto, that, having their fruit unto holiness, they may have the end, eternal life. (Scots Confession, ch. 16, p. 210)

Ethical actions, according to the Westminster formulation, were now anchored in the free will; though they inevitably manifest the divine grace in our life, they serve practical purposes, and since they chasten life, they are pathfinders to eternal life.

Calvinism thus came to be characterized by a free, almost promiscuous and compulsive, exercise of righteousness. This became both its creative genius and its ugliness. The virtues stressed, unfortunately, represented but a narrow range of the full biblical spectrum. Psychosexual and economic values predominated, to the neglect of justice, mercy, and compassion for the poor.

What influence has this moral tradition had on human choices in vitality and suffering, curing and dying? Novelists and social commentators have made much of the influence of Puritan-Presbyterian morality on such health issues as sexuality, sanity, hygiene, and suffering. In general, Presbyterian morality can be defended in that it has created an ethos characterized by honesty, industry, virtue (especially accomplishment), temperance (especially in the Anabaptist form of Calvinism), frugality, and endurance. In social-political ethics this tradition has given much effort to creating the conditions for health, public health, sanitation, preventive medicine, lifestyle discipline, and the like. But in accenting health as achievement it has surely fostered the unfortunate attitude that loss of health in some sense signals moral failure. While in some cases disease does in fact issue from our vicious life-style (for instance, where liver disease arises from alcoholism, lung cancer from smoking, and venereal disease from promiscuity), in another sense this attitude itself has caused much disease and suffering. The person who pares away many of life's pleasures—drinking, laughing, and sensuality among them—may be, as Rabelais would say, prudent and virtuous, but the greater fool. The goal toward which he strives may one day reveal itself to be the grave.

To the medieval and Reformation ideal of the moral person as one who overcomes the world, the flesh, and the devil in divinely spirited existence, the age of Protestant orthodoxy added the ingredients of law, freedom, and conscience. In the famous passage that John Locke took to heart from his Puritan father, it was written:

> God alone is Lord of the conscience, and hath left it free from the doctrines and commandments, of men which are in anything contrary to his Word. . . . So that to believe such doctrines, or to obey such commands out of conscience, is to betray true liberty of conscience; and the requiring of an implicit faith, and an absolute and blind obedience, is to destroy liberty of conscience, and reason also. (Westminster Confession, ch. 20, pp. 215–16)

The great Calvinist philosophers and political sages, Scots, English, and Continental, who formulated the constitutions and bills of rights of the modern nation-states, had this same notion of liberty in mind. They were not committed, as we have tended to think, to an undefined freedom. Conscience was bound to the Word and will of God; no other authority could assume such power. The modern claim that freedom of conscience justifies all manner of private action is the very antithesis of what Locke, Hutcheson, Madison, Witherspoon, and other Calvinist thinkers had in mind.

As we move into the modern world we see this ethic of emancipation moving in the direction of autonomy. Kant defined enlightenment as "man's release from his self-incurred tutelage." *Sapere aude!* "Have courage to use your own reason!" was the motto of the Enlightenment. Tillich went on to claim that autonomy, rather than being chaotic egoism, substituted "universal reason" for "the word of God" as the divine natural law.[10]

In Kant, and in modern moral philosophy in the deontological tradition, the moral law of reason was universalized and seen therefore to be a necessary quality of practical reason. The problem with this, and with other Enlightenment ideology, was that it underestimated human malevolence and the possibility that reason might be misused. Whereas the Calvinist Renaissance and the Puritan creation of our modern Western philosophical and political ethos stressed human depravity and our propensity to misconstrue reason and do wrong, their followers were more optimistic about the human prospect. But following Hume and the French philosophers, the modern states built checks and balances into government because they believed, following biblical anthropology, that man, individual and collective, was not to be trusted. Autonomy ethics, while rightly rejecting heteronomy (the tyranny of another will), failed to sustain theonomous and heteronomous (service of neighbor) ethics because of its naïveté about the reasonableness and goodness of the self.

In an age in which the moral and religious consensus has been shattered, we best sustain the negative checks on moral tyranny, such as conscience and tolerance, which were born in the Calvinist spirit. Barth has argued that the grounding of ethics is not found in politics, philosophy, or human psychology, but in the doctrine of God. The electing grace of God puts us under divine command. Before our self-determination lies the predetermination of God. The ongoing human attempts to reach ethical formulations through reason is part of our primeval propensity to wish to know as God knows "what is good and evil." Though "the grace of God protests against all man-made ethics," it also says yes. Its yes to man is the picture of Adam as upright man, as whole and righteous man given to us in Jesus Christ (*Dogmatics*, II/2, pp. 516–17).

Case Study: Medical Ethics: Bionomy, Homonomy, Theonomy

> God does not believe it odd, that man does not
> believe in God.
> Man believes as best he can, which means, it seems,
> belief in man.
>> (Paddy Chaevsky, *Gideon*)

Biomedical crises, decisions of life and death, test our starting points in ethics. While the temptation in these crises is to affirm self, health, and life, the pull of divine and altruistic perspectives is also felt in such situations.

There are three viable schools of contemporary medical ethics: these might be called bionomous, homonomous, and theonomous approaches. We can behave instinctively, according to biological impulses. We can construct rational, humane systems of ethics. We can seek divine guidance for our decisions. There is good found in each dimension. Each should offer critique and enrichment to the others.

Sociobiology, the study of animal ethology, has recently shed much light on the moral behavior of humans. We are bound to one another, especially in family and society, by bonds and instincts that serve survival, species perpetuation, growth, protection, altruism, and many other values. These virtues are indeed powers supplied by our genetic endowment and evolutionary heritage. We are the only species that willfully threatens itself with extinction. Humans and rats seem obsessed with fratricide. Yet we are also the only species capable of organizing ourselves against ecological extinction. If we can fashion a universal human society, bound together by reciprocity and mutual respect, the divine drama of evolution may be allowed to continue.

This century has produced unprecedented violence: man against himself, his fellow man, and his environment. It has also witnessed the faltering attempts to create world order and to make the good life universally available. The universal Declaration of Human Rights, the United Nations, the World Health Organization, the World Bank, the North-South dialogue— all are old structures that seek to establish a just and humane world order on the basis of reason and ethics. War, torture, oppression, poverty, and disease are not an inevitable or divinely inflicted fate. They are deep, seemingly intractible, but not insoluble problems. The world was not made, or meant to be, the way we have made it. Recognizing God's lordship and our finitude and cohumanity, we can move slowly forward toward that earthly peace the Jew calls "shalom."

Finally, our ethic must always lie open to the transcendent corrective and vision of good. But only a pure, godly, and humanistic faith will do. We cannot baptize human malevolence and injustice by divine sanctions, as we have done since the dawn of history. With Dietrich Bonhoeffer, we must sense the mysterious divine mandate that we are to live in the world without recourse to God but in cohumanity with our fellows. Ethics in the Reformed spirit, then, subtly blends earthiness and transcendence, realism and hope.

Anthropologists Lionel Tiger and Robin Fox have laid before us our current dilemma in ethics. The Renaissance, they have written, celebrated the personality and the individual, yet "robbed humans" of the kind of order in which evil was acknowledged and human energies channeled by a "supervisory abstraction." No such "generous God" now holds our technology in check, as we overcrowd, suffocate, and bomb ourselves.

> Spaceship earth is on its own; so are its humans. . . . If the universal megalopolis that we are building for ourselves can no longer find its unity as the City of God, then it must find it as the City of Man.[11]

Realism is the enduring value in ethics. Realism means responding to reality (the world and God) as it in fact is. When Jesus met the woman at the well (John 4:8–30) he told her "all she ever was" and he received her as a person infinitely precious. A realistic candor from below and a realistic concern from above are the essence of ethics in the human perspective chastened by the transcendent.

HEALING

"All healing is of God," wrote Leslie Weatherhead. "No man has ever healed another. All he has done is to cooperate with God either on the physical, psychological, psychical, or spiritual level of man's personality."[12] If God is the reconciler of life, then healing is not an exclusively physical or spiritual phenomenon; it is a dynamic process that appears at that point where God's perfection interacts with our imperfection. Healing takes place at the intersection of the saving wholeness of our being that is hid with Christ in God within our distressed body and mind. Empirically considered, healing seems to take place "in itself." Antibiotics may be introduced to aid the defensive struggle of the organism against an infection, but no bacteriologist or virologist would ever suggest that the agent was the cure. Similarly, the psychiatrist often watches as a person, perhaps a young person on profound schizophrenic swings, starts to become well. The doctor knows that while her ministrations may have been instrumental to healing, what she is witnessing is a process that has its own power and momentum. This may explain why most disorders, especially mental ones, are cured in approximately the same time and with the same frequency regardless of therapeutic modality. One could say the body heals itself. Hippocrates attributed healing power to nature itself (*via mediatrix naturae*). Most patients, however, experience in illness and recovery not their own therapeutic accomplishment but the presence of a recuperative power greater than themselves.

At the conclusion of Barth's discussion of the ministries of reconciliation, he turned to *Seelsorge*, the cure of souls. This healing activity is directed to the whole person. Barth reminded us to refer to the biblical notion of the "totality of the human being in his personal existence" (*Dogmatics*, IV/3, p. 885). Healing is carried out by every member of the community toward one another. We live with one another as if we are all God's redeemed community. Assuming that we are all children of God, we hold out healing consolation to one another.

> Here in the cure of souls there can and should be confession and with the promise of remission of sins . . . and the invitation to the resultant amendment of life . . . Here in certain extraordinary conditions of emergency and conflict . . . there may be actions analogous to the healings and exorcisms which received such emphasis in the charge to the first disciples. (*Dogmatics*, IV/3, p. 886)

The 1963 Princeton Seminary baccalaureate speaker was Paul Tillich. The title and text of his sermon shocked this class of sophisticated, newly demythologized young theologians: "Heal the Sick, Cast Out Demons."[13] This sermon, which had been delivered first to New York's Union Theological Seminary graduates a few years before, claimed that God had invested the church with special power to heal and cast out demons.

Healing, Tillich said, first requires a candid acknowledgment of our sickness. "Those who are well do not need a physician," said Jesus (Matt. 9:12). The first task of the healing ministry is to remind ourselves that we are not whole, that there is healing grace available, and that the power to conquer the demonic forces that control our lives is at hand. "Evil [sickness] reveals the greatness and the danger of life" (p. 49). The person who can become sick is greater than he who cannot, "who is bound to remain what he is" (p. 49).

Man's life is most open to diseases. For in man's life, more than in any other being, there are divergent trends that must continually be kept in unity. (p. 50)

Christians in the modern age have lost both the courage to confront one another in their illness and the confidence in God's healing spirit. During the early centuries of the Christian era, the exorcism and healing power of the church slowly disappeared. Nursing and invalid care took the place of direct cure. Endurance of suffering was commended in the place of healing. The church that has ceased to risk sickness and even demoniac influences has "little power to heal and to cast out demons" (p. 50). Sickness tears us away from ourselves. It disrupts and disunites our being. In this tearing apart we are drawn to the divine spirit: "no sickness can be healed nor any demon cast out without the reunion of the human spirit with the divine spirit" (p. 52).

Much of our healing does not reach to this level. When Cotton Mather as physician-pastor found his patient-parishioners sick with consumption, he invited them to consider their destiny and the way in which this sickness revealed their neglect and distance from God and provided opportunity for confession and reconciliation.[14] Today, with the exception of psychoanalysis and some wholistic medicine, our concern is often to patch things up temporarily, to mask symptoms. We camouflage the symptoms of allergic hypersensitivity with desensitization shots and antihistamines. This brings relief but may not deal with the underlying problems, which may be genetic, organic, psychosomatic, or some combination of these. We prescribe antihypertensive medications both to mask the symptoms and to offset the deleterious effects of high blood pressure. These, too, may be genetically and biochemically mediated or rooted in anxiety, unresolved guilt, unrealistic expectations, or an inordinate fear of death. We may dish out a chemical or surgical fix instead of dealing with underlying problems. Healing should be sought on the basis of a love for the ailing person in the total fabric of his or her life, when medical symptoms reflect more complex concerns.

Healing in the Reformed Tradition

The Reformed tradition of theology and ethics acknowledges healing as a gift of God entrusted to human implementation. The tradition steers a careful course between the distortions of magic and manipulation on either side of humanly mediated divine healing.

Biblical and primitive wisdom was summarized in the Apocryphal book Ecclesiasticus, or the Wisdom of Jesus the Son of Sirach.

My son, if you have an illness, do not neglect it, but pray to the Lord, and he will heal you. Renounce your faults, amend your way, and cleanse your heart from all sin.

Honor the doctor for his services, for the Lord created him.

The Lord has created medicines from the earth, and a sensible man will not disparage them.

[God] spreads health over the whole world. (Sir. 38:1–12)

Healing blends self-awareness, prevention, and life-style health maintenance; the skill of the physician; the therapy of medicaments—all viewed as manifesting the single healing desire of God.

Prayer and confession is the proper disposition of the psyche that seeks healing. Some intractible illnesses were not remediable even by faith, but only by prayer and fasting (Mark 9:16–29). In the *Didache*, the Way of Life requires that one confess one's faults, unburden one's conscience, and be reconciled to one's brother before health is possible (4:14; cf. Matt. 5:24).

In book 7 of the *City of God* Augustine raised the question of natural powers: whether they should be honored and their power sought in life's adversity. Augustine dealt with the therapeutic powers of the planets and other natural forces and found them impotent. Here Augustine recapitulated an ancient Hebraic thread that counseled against resort to magic, witchcraft, sorcery, and the like in the quest of healing. Augustine argued that it was impossible for demons (mediators of spirit through nature) to come to the aid of persons in reconciliation (healing) because they, too, were slaves of vice (*C.D.* 7.1).

The Sumero-Akkadian and other ancient Oriental religions believed that nature's powers or the gods' beneficence or maleficence could be controlled by incantation, formulas, the wearing of amulets, and so forth. The Hebrews were always tempted to resort to these healing measures and forgot that the Lord was their physician (Exod. 15:26). Even Isaiah placed the diviner on the same plane as the judge and prophet (Isa. 3:2–3). The Deuteronomic law prohibited all magical healing: soothsaying, sorcery, necromancy, enchanting, charming (Deut. 18:10–11). The Levitical law (e.g., Lev. 19:26) and the canon law of late Judaism forcefully condemned all those practices because they identified power in a source alien from God (and were therefore a lie) and honored and worshiped those powers, stealing devotion from God (and were therefore immoral). Paul, in the spirit of the

Old Testament, condemned the magician Bar Jesus as "an enemy of righteousness" (Acts 13:10) and John called the sorcerer a "liar and murderer" (Rev. 9:26).

Yet the practice of magic and supernatural healing persisted (even into our own time). The great church father Origen believed not only in healing but in magical exorcism. If the letters of the name *Jesus* were put in the right order, he said, they had therapeutic value even apart from any association with the Lord himself.[15]

The Middle Ages not only abandoned the healing ministry of the apostolic church but resorted to a wide range of pagan rituals in healing. Fragments of bones and clothes from the saints were said to bear therapeutic power. Shrines, pools, and other holy places became objects of veneration and pilgrimage. Saint Veronica's handkerchief was said to work countless healings and Saint Cuthbert's body did not decompose for seven hundred years as it lay in Durham exuding healing effect.

The Lutheran, and especially Calvinist, Reformation harshly criticized this devotion. Their main objection, of course, was that such obsession gave a false sense of salvation. If indulgences, pilgrimages, and adoration of saints and relics could save and heal, then the doctrine of *sola gratia, sola fide* was wrong. The Puritans were especially critical of these remnants of medieval Catholic indulgence and healing cults. They tore down statues, destroyed all manner of liturgical art and vestments, and broke apart the shrines and relics.

Despite this iconoclasm and its tragic consequences, it is interesting to note that spiritually sensitive medicine continued to be practiced among Calvinist and nonconformist physicians long after medicine had been secularized among the establishment. The journals of Calvinist physicians who practiced in England, Holland, France, or Germany in the seventeenth century reveal a responsiveness to divine healing as an accompaniment to their empirical medicine. Their diaries display an interest in the interpretation of divine etiology (what caused this and what does it mean?). They found the experiences of birth and death fraught with theological significance. They therefore imbued these experiences with ministries of spiritual meaning. Similarly, mental disorders, melancholia, and the like were interpreted and treated theologically, an approach not found in orthodox (Anglican, Roman Catholic, and Lutheran) medicine.

The enduring spirit of Calvinism on the issues of healing is an acknowledgment of the empirical medical arts (medicine, pharmacy, surgery, psychiatry, and nursing) as the chosen instrumentality of divine healing. God alone heals, and he does it through these ministries. When the healing arts are spiritualized into magic they are condemned; when they are reduced to human manipulations, they are similarly condemned—healing is excellent human science rendered in careful technique against the backdrop of the therapeutic spirit of God.

Miracles and Faith Healing: At this point it is necessary to deal with the questions of miracles, exorcisms, and faith healing. These phenomena have not been condemned in the churches' support of the secular healing arts; they are considered positive features of the Spirit's reconciling work at integral points in the total healing enterprise. As such they offer much difficulty, embarrassment, and misunderstanding to doctors, nurses, and pastors today, as they have in previous centuries.

The grand question of miracles, as C. S. Lewis has reminded us, is the question of the resurrection. If that root miracle has indeed occurred, other healings surely are possible. Signs and wonders (*semeia* and *terata*) were occurrences in the New Testament that evidenced the power of God (*dynamis*). Jesus had healing *dynamis* on his hands (Mark 6:5) as did Paul (Gal. 3:5; Rom. 15:1).

As we survey the Bible in its presentation of miracles, we see that life itself (Gen. 2:4–24), and its conception (Gen. 4:25, 17:15–21; Matt. 1:20), were miracles. The concentration of miraculous healings around the Christ event can be attributed first to the unusual spiritual power that was found in the Savior, second to the expectation and readiness to be healed found in those who came to him, and third to the general acceptance of healing miracles in Judaic and Hellenistic culture (Aesclepius in France, Strabo in Rome). The attempts to rationalize the miracles, such as saying that there were stones on Lake Galilee or that the people had concealed their bread, do not help. All we can say is that God, as we have come to know him, is capable of suspending or altering nature's working if he chooses. After all, he started it and sustains it. He is sovereign over nature. We also know that faith is an awesome force in human experience. Given the great range of unpredictability, spontaneity, and possibility in human experience, and given the very limited knowledge we have of cause and effect, of natural process, indeed, of reality itself, there is a great opportunity for what can be called the miraculous to occur.

The enduring teaching of the Reformed faith is that all of life is a miracle, since it proceeds from the reconciling purposes of God. The healing arts are extolled throughout Hebrew and Christian history as provisions of God. All healing proceeds from God's spirit, and occasions for miraculous intervention in the course of nature are in his hands. God's will for us is to receive his life, be his reconciling agents in health and in sickness, in life and at death. All of these experiences are provisions of his will for us. Jesus prayed that his life might be spared (Matt. 26:39). Paul asked for relief from his "thorn in the flesh" (2 Cor. 12:7). Neither miracle, neither prayer, was granted. The larger purpose of God moved in another direction.

Case Study: Faith Healing Houses and Hospices

The persistent yearning of the human spirit for miracles and the equally persistent mind of new science to deny spirit and miracles has led us to create two health-care systems. The secular, scientific system tends to body-machines with only the glorious power of technological medicines. The houses of healing (like Oral Roberts Medical Center in the Calvinistic Bible belt) and hospices (like Saint Helen's and Saint Christopher's in Britain's scientific heartland of London and Oxford) are efforts of the counterculture. In the first type of institution, manipulation of body and mind passes for total-person therapy. In the latter, humane, even spiritual ministry, is paramount and scientific medicine may be deemphasized. What is needed surely is a renewed understanding of God as reconciling physician, then a new concept of person as a whole being in whom all health and disease is a mind-body-spirit experience. Finally, a new concept of healing must emerge that celebrates both the material arts of medicine and a spiritual and moral sensitivity in interpreting the source of disease, effecting cure, and making endurance meaningful.

CARING

When everyone is somebodee, / Then no one's anybody. (Gilbert and Sullivan)

Since injustice is an abomination to God, we should render to each man what belongs to him. (Rom. 13:7) (Calvin, *Institutes*, 2.8, p. 408)

God wills that there be equality among us. This means that no one should have too little and no one too much. (Calvin, *Commentaries on Second Corinthians*)

God has been described as reconciler of humanity. By this we understand that he has drawn all people to himself, as on the cross he uplifted Christ from the earth in sacrificial death. This atonement has also created a new community among people where previously prevailing distinctions, hierarchies, and order no long hold sway (Gal. 3:28–29). Indeed, in the liberating Messiah (Luke 4:18–19), good news is proclaimed to the poor, and the oppressed are set free. Mary's Magnificat, recalling the song of Hannah in the Old Testament, is the charter of freedom for all people:

> He has torn imperial powers from their thrones,
> but the humble have been lifted high.
> The hungry he has satisfied with good things.
> The rich sent empty away.
>   (Luke 1:52–53)

When it comes to concern for the poor, the sick, and needy, an even stronger quality of God's character makes itself known. He is not only the reconciler, but the avenger of wrong and the advocate of the needs of the oppressed. Justice (Hebrew: *sedek*; Greek: *dikaion*) is not just impartiality or giving each person his due. It is the positive disposition toward persons in need. Justice, in this theological sense, is God's righteous energy to maintain, secure, heal, and edify. He positively attacks those who would deprive or harm his children. He enlists his children to raze the structures of injustice and raise new sources of care. He rewards the efforts of those who struggle to humanize the conditions, structures, and institutions of life. He punishes evil and rewards good. He delivers from enemies (Ps. 5:8), including pestilence, exposure, and need (Ps. 91:1–7). God pursues the course of the hungry, the sick, the prisoner, the blind, the orphan, the poor and needy (Amos 2:6). Although we humans seek to perpetuate the structures of privilege and injustice, these are always being overturned by the reconciling, justice-bearing spirit of God. As the nature of God as reconciler makes its demand on us as care givers to one another, we are saved from the injustices of sentimental paternalism and mechanical dispensation. In health care, these two risks are great blights on what should be the most sensitive arena of human charity.

As we view our health-care system today we find it a sorry mixture of paternalism and impersonalism, inflicting not only neglect but positive harm on persons. Even though we pour roughly 10 percent of our gross national product into health care, the breakdown in the system is painfully obvious. The irony of the situation is that caring people are found throughout the system: there is a spark of human feeling and altruism in the most hardened physician. He certainly would not endure the many years of rigorous training simply for a lucrative and prestigious career; if he wanted wealth, surely he would have entered law, real estate, or business. Nurses, too, are a compassionate lot. Even though it often seems that they are clock-punchers, dispensers of orders, and administrators running activities on the hospital wards from their distant computer screens at the end of the hall, caring alone explains their long-suffering work for meager wages. The same can be said for other health workers, administrators, or trustees of institutions. No other sector of our society so compels our caring and philanthropic instincts as the health-care system.

Then what has gone wrong? In the first place, the reconciling God has been replaced by another god: success, growth, and profits. Secondly, our view of man has changed from one where we esteem persons as unique, precious, and mysterious selves to one where we view them as body-machines, as exquisite collages of organs and tissues. Medical theory and practice continue to perpetuate the myth that diseases are simple and specific phenomena amenable to isolation, diagnosis, and specific therapy, and that therapies can be localized to diseased organs, systems, or syndromes. This specific definition of disease and therapy is slowly breaking down as we understand more about disorders and cures, but in the meantime we disgrace ourselves by talking about "the liver in room 20," "the heart in room 32," "the gall-bladder in the O.R."

Finally, and most grievously, the constant weight of attending the sick, suffering, and dying has taken its toll. A generation of care-givers who lack the staying power, sympathy, and compassion that a religious faith used to supply now begin to crack under the demands of working amid pain, anguish, stench, anger, and abuse. Persons press through the health-care system today in staggering numbers, presenting a dizzying and draining array of symptoms and needs. But even when the number of care-givers is adequate to patient numbers (as the ratio of four to one at a famed cancer hospital), care seems routine, rushed, impersonal; healing is surely impeded as the "self" of the patient is thus reduced and humiliated. To survive when personal resources are being sucked dry, to become once more the comforter and healer of those suffering persons, health professionals must reassess the nature of "care" itself: that it is a divine grace received in piety and nurtured under serious spiritual discipline.

Paul Ramsey has used the word "care" to describe the set of moral obligations and opportunities that we hold toward the sick. When we ask the moral question "what should we do" in a concrete medical situation, we must first ask:

> What singular deed or design of ours is most likely to embody or convey care or respect for human life? We ask, will this or that procedure care for the patient more? Or we ask, will this or that research design be productive of the more significant benefit for the ongoing community of medical care?[16]

As T. S. Eliot wrote, there is a time to care and a time not to care. Care often requires giving up, choosing one instead of another, even inflicting pain. An example of this strange kind of care is the new cancer treatment in which chemotherapy has devastating systemic effects on the body: this is carried out in the hope of so destroying the malignant cells that the body's own immune system will take over and check any further development of the tumor.

Sometimes care requires comfort and consolation. Sometimes it requires severe measures of surgery or confrontational psychotherapy. Sometimes care requires counsel and exhortation. Sometimes care requires choosing between two lives (as in abortion) or saving some and not all (as in triage). In these difficult situations, we may turn to the wisdom of the Reformed tradition.

Caring in the Reformed Tradition

The earliest moral structures provided constraints on maleficence, which, by implication, encouraged beneficence. The Code of Hammurabi (ca. 1800 B.C.) and other ancient Near Eastern legal and moral codes prescribed penalties for harms done and generally concentrated on negative sanctions rather than positive incentives to care. In the Old Testament, the positive side of this ancient tradition was made central. The golden rule was lifted out of the ancient notion of revenge and retaliation and made into a positive imperative:

> You shall not seek revenge, or cherish anger . . .
> You shall love your neighbor as a man like yourself.
> I am the Lord. (Lev. 19:18)

Here, beneficence and respect that visits no harm or injury on another acknowledge the divine presence in oneself and in the other. Injuring and killing were seen as suicidal and blasphemous, an assault on God himself. Benevolence, a caring disposition toward others that actively promotes their good, is a response to the divine life in us. God demands *hesed*, righteous, positive justice and concern for others, rather than words and rituals (Hos. 6:6; Mic. 6:8).

The great contribution of the Bible and the Jewish people to world history is to introduce us to God as the tender-hearted lover of his creation and its people. God is introduced as the maker of a covenant (a reciprocal arrangement for life). From his side, abiding care, mercy, and forgiveness are given without condition. Our proper response is to love Yahweh, walk in his ways

(Deut. 10:12, 11:22, 19:9), and keep his commandments (Exod. 20:6; Deut. 5:10). We do not care for others because we want to or like to, or because it pays off or returns to us (Kant). No hedonistic or utilitarian justification matters. We love because God loves us (1 John 4:19).

God is love. We know it because Christ depicts God for us and his life is love: deep, searching, sacrificing love. God loved the world so much that he gave his only son (John 3:16). In the New Testament we find the language of love prevailing in the Johannine and, to a somewhat lesser extent, Pauline, literature. That the synoptic Gospels and Acts use the word little can be explained by the urgency of the Markan and synoptic purpose: to plea for repentance and righteousness as the kingdom shatters this world and hastens it toward its consummation. (Jesus did, however, forcefully recapitulate the Old Testatment command to "love the Lord your God. . . . love, your neighbor as yourself" [Mark 12:30–31; Matt. 19:19]).

Once the church had settled in, the imperatives of mutual care and concern for the world became more central. "See how they love each other," was the observation of a critical onlooker (John 15:12; Rom. 13:8). When the *Didache* was formulated as a teaching instrument for the apostolic church (A.D. 100), it began its instructions with a description of the "way of life" as opposed to the "way of death." The command to love God and the neighbor, along with the golden rule, were the first and foremost elements in this creed. That love is placed in such a central position reveals how important this concern was to the early church.

> There are two ways, one of Life and one of Death, and there is much difference between the two ways. The way of Life is this: firstly, thou shalt love God who made thee. Secondly, thou shalt love thy neighbor as thyself: and whatsoever thou wouldst not have done to thyself, do not thou either to another. (*Didache* 1:1)

The Acts of the Apostles describe the primitive communism of the early church. Property was held in common and the community looked after the needs of its own near and far. In Paul, the controlling virtue of the moral life is *agapē* (1 Cor. 13). In the apostolic church this becomes the basis of the love ethic, finally developed fully in Augustine's exposition of *caritas* (cf. *Confessions* 12.30). For Augustine, *caritas serviens* became the essence of Christian living. This style of existence, built on the *kenosis* chapter of Philippians (2:5 ff.) and the humility extolled in the Sermon on the Mount, became the archetype for the mendicant-service orders of the church and the *imitatio Christi* piety of the Middle Ages. Hospitals, hospices, and houses for the sick and needy flourished all over the Christian Roman Empire because of this spirit.

A breach then occurred in patristic and medieval thought. Although most of the late fathers agreed that inequality, distinction, and hierarchy did not exist in the original creation, the Fall initiated a state of dissociation in the social fabric that allowed aggression and aggrandizement to separate the human family. The moral commitment of caring shifted from a sense of natural belonging to one another to the thought that the rich were morally obligated to give alms liberally and charitably and to care paternalistically for the disadvantaged.[17] This misconstrual of *caritas* as obligatory or manipulative act frequently occurs in the tradition and today underlies such barbarous concepts as "health-care delivery."

Caring seen in terms of administration and power, a concept that emerged in the modern world, has ancient roots. When John Wycliffe composed his treatise *De civili domino* in Oxford in 1374, he proposed that only the Christian righteous could hold lordship over others, for they were trustworthy in beneficence. Otherwise, all good things were to be held in common, since in the state of grace the whole world belonged to every person. Since this evidently was not the prevailing situation, the godly civil order should administer the common goods so that their benefit accrued to all.[18]

Wycliffe and, later, Luther believed that the caring and provident principles that ordered the divine reign in the kingdom of God should be appropriated as much as possible in the civil order. Much in the spirit of Wycliffe, Luther claimed, "A Christian is perfectly free lord of all, subject to more, and perfectly dutiful servant of all, subject to all."[19] Care was thus lifted out of the nexus of personal compassion and neighborly assistance into the realm of institutional care.

The modern world has witnessed the proliferation of politically created institutions for the care of the sick and dying. Even hospitals that originated in a religious charter have, for the most part, become bureaucratic business enterprises. Conflicts arise out of the two antithetical kinds of human contracts that are at work: the healer-patient relationship is, of course, a voluntary association based on reciprocity, trust, and patient consent; the corporation-client association is based on power, order, and patient compliance.[20]

In our recent experience, this configuration of caring has led on the one side to the desire to effect structural change, to develop more humane "deliver care" in "humanized institutions."[21] Schubert Ogden, writing in the same spirit of liberation theology, has argued that "God's own emancipating work consists in meeting this deeper creaturely need for a world in which one can freely determine one's own destiny in solidarity with one's fellow creatures."[22]

Gustavo Gutierrez has said, "The poor [and the sick] person is a by-product of the system in which we live . . . his poverty is not the call for a generous act which will alleviate his misery, but rather a demand for building a different social order."[23] In this new mentality, care involves the assertion of rights to the common resource, the advocacy of the needy in the public forum, and the creation of institutions that are more responsive to concerns for self-determination and human solidarity based not on paternalistic beneficence but on cohumanity.

The spirit of the Reformed tradition fosters a strong commitment to human advocacy and a call for comprehensive and edifying care for persons. Such care does not serve the giver; it serves the power, health, and self-determination of the recipient. After giving a person fish to eat, the giver teaches him to fish. At the same time the Protestant spirit is not one that tends toward radical individualism. Calvinism recognizes that we are all mortal and morbidly ill. We are given to mutual care in covenant communities because we are all caught in the tragedy and delight of life together. God in Christ lives in the midst of human crisis, inviting those to whom he has given strength to aid the weakness of others until that equation is reversed. Parents care for their children until, in the maturity of time, the child cares for the parent. That simple biological phenomenon provides the paradigm for human caring.

The kind of care required today in the realm of health and illness is both profoundly personal yet structural, in that it must genuinely convey freedom and power. Caring must occur over backyard fences, in supermarkets, in bars, and in barbershops. In all the places where we routinely traffic with one another we must develop the grace to hear pain, to allow it to surface and fully expose its effect, then to attend to the tasks of healing.

The professional and community resources of caring for physical, mental, familial, and environmental disturbance must be enhanced. To do this, the churches and synagogues (which first received the commission to stand by those in need) must reenter the health-care system, offering that powerful service they can best provide.

Since the church possesses unique engagement with people at critical points in their lives (e.g., birth, marriage, poverty, suffering, dying), it should develop congregation-based clinics to provide the following health care services:

(1) Family-planning counseling to help couples make decisions about

bearing children, transmitting genetic traits, and the like, and especially to help deal with the inevitable value questions.

(2) Pregnancy, conception, and birth counseling: dealing with the issues of fetal anaylsis, abortion, conception control, areas so fraught with moral concerns, and needing support and forgiveness.

(3) The church has a marvelous entrée to the life of the young adults as they contemplate, prepare for, and actually enter the marriage relationship. Since biomedical and emotional needs intertwine so deeply with the moral and spiritual dimensions of life, care within the church context would be most helpful.

(4) The churches have great resources to serve people at crisis points. For the terminally ill, the churches could develop extensive ministries of preparation, home care, and companionship. This might obviate the disgrace of allowing so many to die in intensive-care units in modern technological hospitals, surrounded by impersonal machines, at incredible expense.

The majestic Norman cathedral in Durham, England, displays a large brass knocker on the great main door. In the Middle Ages, if someone was able to reach that knocker and gain entrance, he would be offered sanctuary and safe passage abroad. The church could again serve people in their life experiences by providing confidentiality and protection. What better way could there be to expend the great financial and personal wealth that exists in the twentieth-century church and synagogue?

Case Study: Caring with Scarce Resources

An advisory committee to the National Institute of Health is charged with monitoring a national study to assess the efficacy of a blood-cleansing procedure called plasma phoresis. This procedure is used for numerous ailments, including arthritis and severe lupus nephritis. It is a very costly treatment that perhaps will benefit many thousands if it proves efficacious. It is a medical resource, like organ replacement and transplantation and neonatal intensive care, that holds the prospect of benefiting many persons, but at costs that the society may not be able to bear. How does one make personal and policy judgments of this type in the light of Reformed ethical tradition?

The following guidelines would seem to emerge from the preceding discussion on caring:

(1) Emphasis should be placed on preventing illness and staying well rather than on attempting rescue at a late stage. Although dramatic intervening medicine does much for the paternalistic self of modern medicine in its mission of mercy, the real needs of people are best served by activities

that keep them well. If the health of a society is attributable in only 6 percent to the medical system and in 94 percent to the systems of sanitation, life-style, fundamental research in human biology, environment, industry, education, and the like, then these are the efforts that should receive health-care dollars.[24]

(2) A system that disallows merit criteria for entry and in which ability to pay does not play a part is in keeping with the Reformed ethic. If triage choices must be made, we should stand aside, seeing this occasion as an opportunity to emulate Christ, who laid down his life for his friends (John 15:11–15). If we must make decisions for a group, an impartial procedure, such as lottery, is most just.

(3) The practice of highly personal, individualized caring must be fostered within our great impersonal systems. When persons are treated as special individuals and not as numbers or cases, there usually emerges a surprising coincidence between what is available and what persons really need. Calvin understood this world as an abundantly provident resource in which God had foreseen every need in our life. Indeed, he does far more for us than we are able to conceive (Eph. 3:20). In ethical situations in hospitals, I've observed that most often there is an exact coincidence between what people want in health, life, and death and what the "care system" is able to provide. This coincidence is found in Puritan simplicity or in Augustine's grace of having what we want and wanting what we have.

Some of the most perplexing quandries of what it means to care are present in the realm of medical choices. To help us in these moments we can only turn to those deep insights of justice and mercy, of conscience and forgiveness, of grace and acceptance, that we receive in faith.

DYING

The Apostle Paul, who had built many tents and knew well that each eventually collapsed or wore out, yearned for a dwelling that would stand forever. He wanted to die and be with Christ. Yet he recognized that he had yet work to do: for the sake of his friends he chose to "stay" in this life to "stand by you all to help you forward and . . . add joy to your faith" (Phil. 1:21–26). In the fullness of God's time, with his service to his friends and for his Lord completed, Paul would joyfully embrace that death by which he gained eternal life with Christ.

Death is God's reward for a life fully and rightly lived: "Come, enter and possess the kingdom that has been ready for you since the world was made" (Matt. 25:34). But we protest that few persons die "in the fullness of time," their talents developed, their goals realized, their cup of happiness full. The point has been made in discussing suffering: Why must a child die from teratogenic injury or acute leukemia? Why was my eighteen-year-old cousin run over as he changed his flat tire, or my friend's seventeen-year-old sweetheart thrown off her bicycle as she rode to visit him? Such deaths—any death that robs us of a warm presence dearly loved—seem "premature," "unnatural," and "untimely," and we seem to be the victims of a capricious, even malevolent, world order. As Kent cries:

> As flies to wanton boys, are we to the gods,
> They kill us for their sport.
> > (*King Lear*, IV, 37–38)

When Florence Dombey asks about her dead young brother, "Why was he born?" the question stings long after the easy replies about the quality of time or the value of "exerting oneself" have faded away.[25]

The scales of justice totter precariously: some deaths come too late, more mockery of Cleopatra's "injurious gods." Augustine once wrote that there was no death in the world by which someone did not stand to profit; the archdeacon of Barchester lost his chance for the bishopric because his ailing father did not die while their family friend was still prime minister.[26] The literary examples pale before the personal ones. "I pray constantly that God will let me die," my once beautiful and fiercely independent aunt said, echoing the misery of many. With countless dollars and tears, we tend the bedridden forms of the once-human, still living.

> . . . then is it sin
> To rush into the secret house of death
> Ere death dare come to us?
> > (*Antony and Cleopatra*,
> > IV, xiii, 81–83)

Some would answer, no sin, only mercy.

The Calvinist faith, however, will not accept the idea that some deaths come too soon and others too late. While it is true that murder is an evil and blasphemous act, even murder and war do not thwart God's prerogative, as Blackstone proposed in his summary of British law (suicides rush into God's presence "uncalled for"). God's will comprehends every death. Not a sparrow falls without his leave (Matt. 10:29).

Every life, every exigency of every life, the beginning and conclusion of every life, is embraced in God's purpose. Does this mean that we do not fasten our seatbelts when we drive? Does predestinarian confidence embolden us to live more carelessly and threaten our health? Surprisingly, Calvinist culture does not favor this kind of resignation and abandon. If anything, this theological spirit stimulates a rigorous stewardship of life and a consciousness of responsibility, in which we act as if everything depended on us.

A wide range of questions in philosophy and ethics hinges on our normative concept of death. The questions of the definition of death (brain criteria or whole body), of prolonging life, or terminating treatment, of aiding death by either active or passive euthanasia, and of suicide are just a few of the issues. Similarly, a spectrum of theological questions can only be explained in the light of biological and medical knowledge. Can we talk of the death of the brain, the mind, the soul? Does clinical experience teach us anything about immortality? In bringing pastoral care to the dying, do we tell the truth about diagnosis and prognosis? Is hope crushed when a person learns of his impending death?

Another treatise on death and dying, on the stages of dying, or on the stages of life after death is not required. These books abound, even in airport shops next to *Hustler* magazine. Death and dying is the pornography of our time.[27] What may prove helpful is a discussion of how the Calvinist spirit in secular culture has created an ethos that shapes the way we approach, individually and collectively, the experience of death. We may then hold over against this secular spirit a review of the theological substance of this tradition that will help us make personal decisions as well as form the fundamental visions and values that will wisely guide the course of medical policy and institutional health care. Such a review of ethical teaching will help us bring a corrective critique to the secular tradition, which runs the risk of excess, even harm, when it is cut loose, as it now is, from its religious moorings.

Charles Webster, director of the Wellcome Institute of the History of Medicine in Oxford, has shown that the Puritan spirit contributed decisively to the emergence of modern biomedical science. In *The Great Instauration* he also shows how the commitment to prolong life emerged within this same ethos. Francis Bacon, whose mother was a devout Puritan, established a road map for the scientific revolution with his two books: *Advancement of Learning* and *Novum Organum*. In these studies he offered not only the destination points but also the route for the journey. Medicine, he argued, has from time immemorial been concerned with the Hippocratic mandate to prevent illness and cure disease. Now the empirical method (corresponding to Puritan firsthand religious experience) and modern technological skill bring an even nobler purpose into view: that of prolonging life. Enamored, as were many of his age, with the intricate mechanical workings of the human body, Bacon believed that the ancient curses of disease and debility (perhaps even death?) might one day be overcome. The Puritan hope was based on the belief that the long dark ages of travail (the medieval world of Catholic society and Galenic medicine) were coming to a close. The millennium was being born, and from these birth pangs a new achievement of life and health would, in the providence of God, arrive.

In the late Middle Ages death was viewed as a warrior-enemy stalking the lives of men. A dying person put down shield and sword, for the battle had already been fought and won: Christ brought one across. The final crossing of that great pilgrim Mr. Valiant-For-Truth, is the final stage of a pilgrimage that has been marked by repeated tests, challenges, and struggles.

> Then said he, I am going to my fathers, and tho' with great difficulty I am got hither, yet now I do not repent me of all the trouble I have been at to arrive where I am. My sword I give to him that shall succeed me in my pilgrimage, and my courage and skill to him that can get it. My marks and scars I carry with me, to be a witness for me that I have fought his battles who will now be my rewarder. When the day that he must go hence was come, many accompanied him to the riverside, into which as he went he said, "Death, where is thy sting?" And as he went down deeper he said, "Grave, where is thy victory?" So he passed over, and all the trumpets sounded for him on the other-side.[28]

His weapons and skills, honed in the quest, are passed on to his successors, who will continue the struggle and the search.

The Christian faith sets in motion two impulses in the human spirit as it confronts the experience of death. The first is the spirit of resistance. Sin brought death into the world. If death is a judgmental force, we are then inspired to resist it and seek to overcome it. In the Middle Ages death was personified as specific deaths. War, the plagues, and hunger were specific diabolic powers that fought to tear life away from our bodies. The modern world sustains this mythology by breaking deaths down into a spectrum of diseases: septic death, cardiac and pulmonary arrest, sudden neurologic crisis. Within the broad categories there are the specific diseases that were given ontologic status in the nineteenth century. Pneumonia, tuberculosis, and cancer were specific deaths. Fighting deaths and overcoming them was defeating a devil. The minister of health in the African republic Cameroon confessed to me at a World Health Organization meeting that his country was in a quandry. The final eradication of small pox left an entire priest-hood and religion in his country hanging because this culture had been solely committed to appeasing and thereby resisting the "smallpox god": as long as sanctuaries remained, priests enacted their rituals, and people brought proper sacrifices, the smallpox god would not bring pestilence. Now, with the practice of vaccination, the cult had been rendered redun-dant. The same psychology is found in the medical conquest of deaths. When one death is vanquished, the sect (with its priests, researchers, and clinicians) must quickly move to another or become obsolete. Right now dentists are developing the knowledge and technology of making their ser-vices unnecessary by emphasizing prevention rather than dental treatment.

The positive side of this resistance to death is love for life. Whereas death was a release during the ages of the plagues—"Vex not his ghost: O, let him pass!" (*King Lear*, V, iii, 315)—in ages of affluence and health we enjoy vitality and are reluctant to give up without a fight. In Tevye's words from *Fiddler on the Roof*, we are so happy we don't realize how miserable we are. The "gray revolution" in the Western world is the protest of a genera-tion that has been provided the blessing of getting old (by medicine, public health, social welfare), but, because of retirement laws or housing patterns, has not been allowed to express that new measure of time meaningfully.

The second impulse born of the divine spirit is that of accepting, even welcoming, death. If the idea of death as an enemy is the Hebraic and Pau-line legacy, very early, as early as the Gospel of John, a mood of anticipa-tion, even desire, is created. In the Persian and Hellenistic world views, where a negation of matter prevailed, a view emerged that this body was a prison for the immortal soul. It is a cocoon, a bird cage, an outer garment, that one day will open and fall away, releasing the pure divine soul to its home. This view of death obviously appealed to the early church, which lived constantly under the threat of impending death. The thought that the body and soul were distinct and separable entities had precedent throughout the ancient Eastern and Western worlds. It was also empirically sensible. When a person died, it appeared that something had gone out of him. Just as exsanguinating quickly led to collapse and exhaustion, so other deaths seemed to be an exhaustion or extraction of the spirit.

Psychodynamically, these two impulses form a dialectic in the human consciousness. Freud called them life and death instincts, or "loves" (*Le-benslust, Todesliebe*). The one serves individual survival by stimulating the creature to avoid danger and to propagate. The other serves species survival by assuring that life will be relinquished to another generation by one's departure. Similarly, religious traditions have warned against overly craving life, so that one cannot relinquish it, and against overly despising life, so that one cannot perpetuate it. Reluctant submission to death in its good time is the course of wisdom. Its "good time" is when life has had a chance for fulfillment and contribution, when second and third generations are pressing from below, and when one's powers have waned so that the *joi de vivre* is gone. One is then "full of years" and passes gracefully (Job 42:17; Gen. 15:15).

Death and Immortality in the Reformed Tradition

The most ancient traditions spoke of death as an experience to be approached with reluctant acceptance. As they grew old and feeble, the Eskimo knew that their time had come and they were pushed off on an ice block (with their reluctant consent, we trust). The migrating tribes would periodically pass through turbulent, rushing rivers, where it was anticipated that some would be washed away. In old African mythology the gods had given life and breath to people. They enjoyed it so much that they refused to return to their maker. The gods then introduced death into the world to bring back their children. Throughout world mythology there is the thought that death has intruded into life either as a punishing act of the gods or as some measure to ensure the return and recycle of life.

The fundamental law of the Noachian covenant is the proscription of murder. This prohibition is seen almost universally in terms of intratribal fratricide. To kill one's own brother is the primal crime that leaves its mark on the human brow. Killing of other people as a defensive act or in protection of one's own livelihood or property is, of course, condoned. The force of ancient Near Eastern Babylonian, Sumerian, and Egyptian laws on murder is seen when we realize the intent of these laws. When humans passed into the wanderer-gatherer epoch of their history, their paramount aim was to survive, to eat, and to preserve the integrity of their own small tribe. When civilization began and communities and cities were formed, the older instincts had to be sublimated into more cooperative patterns of living. Sanctions were now imposed for acts of violence. Only retaliatory and defensive acts of violence were tolerated; indeed, they were required.

The Bible is a drama of human life and death in an unfolding story bounded at both ends by the symbol of the tree of life (Gen. 2:9; Rev. 22:14). God is sole possessor of the power over life and death. Though man would like to take this knowledge and power into his own hands, God retains this authority. In the Old Testament we find the idea that God himself struggles to gain power over death. In earliest Judaism *sheol* is the shadowy abode of death where the human call for God is no longer heard and where praise is impossible. Death was in one sense an abandonment of mankind, as the Gilgamesh Epic stated: When the gods created humanity, they established death for mankind, they kept life in their own hands.[29] To be ill was to be abandoned to *sheol*; recovery was victory over death (Ps. 9:13). The gods were called upon to rescue one from the "net of death" (Ps. 18:6, 116:3). The Hebrew God slowly emerged as one who could enter the realm of death and even hold sway there (Hos. 13:14). Ultimately, God was pictured as being engaged in a struggle with the power of death. The giver and keeper of life had to absorb this power over death to perfect his purpose (2 Cor. 5:4). In this sense the vocation of Jesus Christ can be seen as a final completion of God's victory over the force of death. In apocalyptic Judaism, world history comes to be divided into two aeons. There is the present age in which we are living (*aiōn houtos*). In this age, strife and death reign, and the struggle of God for victory over the power of evil and death is still incomplete. In the coming age (*aiōn mellōn*), these hostile powers will be overcome and God will reign in life with his children. Much of the theology of late Judaism, even from the exilic Prophets and Psalms, anticipated this messianic victory over the powers of darkness and death. Death as power is founded in man's resistance to God, in sin, and in the arrival of demonic powers on earth. Adam's Fall made the human story one of "destiny to death" (Tillich). Eventually the locus of God's power over death came to be conceived in terms of bodily resurrection. Death could not be overcome; it was now ingrained into the universe. Now it would be overwhelmed by resurrection after death.

The appearance of Christ, and his resurrection from the dead, is cast in the light of this Hebraic tradition. We know very little of the factual details of Jesus' resurrection. He had given advanced notice; at least the Evangelists remembered him saying that he would die and in three days rise again. What we do know is that a vivid experience occurred for Jesus' disciples very shortly after his death. They were surprisingly regathered after it was quite certain they had finally disbanded in despair. They were empowered with a message and an energy that was to change the world. In the apostolic preaching, they came to believe that God had taken the side of the crucified one, had decisively endorsed this crucifixion-resurrection act, and had made it the decisive event in his redemption of the world (Acts 2:24, 3:5, 4:10, 5:31).

The primitive Christian community believed that the cross had become God's decisive victory over the powers of death (Ps. 110; 1 Cor. 15:25; Heb. 10:13). The humiliation of the cross had been to good effect, for now God had "highly exalted him" (Acts 5:31; Phil. 2:9). The power of this "last enemy" (1 Cor. 15:26) had been broken. Jesus had broken the root cause of death, human sin. Death no longer had power or control (Rom. 6:7 ff.). Believers now knew victory over death as they experienced victory over sin. In baptism we die and rise with Christ (Rom. 6:3; Gal. 6:14; Col. 2:20). The newness of life in which sin is denied sway and righteousness and immortality are given life is called "eternal life" (John 3:36).

Life, no longer grounded in sin, now defiant of death, is moral life. Participation in the expiatory death of Christ is now to contend boldly with Christ against the continuing force of the powers of death. Discipleship is fellowship in suffering (Mark 8:34–35). The martyr (witness) is one who gives his life in Christ's name (Mark 13:13; Acts 15:26). The witness to Christ was one who "shed his blood in godly service to man" (Acts 22:20; Rev. 2:13, 12:11). Later, the New Testament takes up the theme of Christ's death controlling our living through humility (Phil. 2:5 ff.), endurance (Heb. 12:1 ff.), patience (I Pet. 2:20 ff.), and love (John 15:13). That we are to die to ourselves and live to God and one another becomes the basis of the *ars moriendi* and *ars vivendi* of the early church. In holy living and holy dying we prepare to pour out our life unto death, as we contend with Christ against the "principalities and powers" that still unleash terrible force in this world (Eph. 6:12). It is also a preparation for death, as we conform our body and soul more and more to Jesus' death and resurrection.

The church of the second and third centuries struggled with its definition of *resurrectio carnis*. In the old Roman Creed, the Apostles Creed, and all other early Christian literature, the doctrine of the resurrection of the flesh, in distinction to the immortality of the soul, was affirmed.

Augustine took the suggestive threads of life-and-death theology found in the Old and the New Testament and in the early church fathers and wove them into a coherent and colorful tapestry. His presentation of the Christian picture of life and death, of heaven and hell, would dominate the popular imagination for a thousand years. In the Middle Ages the drama turned into a torturous and lurid apocalypse. When Dante's *Divine Comedy* represented the sublime drama of death and redemption, it was reiterating Augustine's story. Even the gentle Pusey, the nineteenth-century philosopher who, with Newman, began the Oxford movement (and in whose Oxford library this chapter is being written), was compelled by the Augustinian vision of heaven and hell:

> This, then, is the first outward suffering of the damned that they are purged, steeped in a lake of fire. O woe, woe, woe!... You know the fierce, intense, burning heat of a furnace, how it consumes in a moment

anything cast into it. Its misery to the damned shall be that they feel it, but cannot be consumed by it.[30]

It is easy to overdramatize the themes that Augustine tried to portray in his doctrine of heaven and hell. Augustine had seen the tragedy of personal life in his own desperate search for delight and meaning. He had studied the sublime wisdom of philosophers and rhetoricians. He had seen the transience and fragility of world history as he watched the vandals sack Rome. Life would be living death, he believed, were it not for the pivotal event of Christ's coming into our humanity and into our history. The picture that the Evangelists and Paul painted provides a true portrait of God, his world, and his plan because the Gospels and Epistles have, in Christ, become the Word of God. There is no satisfaction of happiness in mortal existence, Augustine wrote. The philosophers have sought felicity in wisdom and justice, in pleasure and renunciation, but all the schools—Platonic, Epicurean, and Stoic, indeed, all of human wisdom—had not found happiness on the temporal plane.

We also know, said Augustine, that death is judgment. We are all called to account for our life by the God who made us. In the *City of God* (20.5) he recited all the Old and New Testament texts which disclosed that we shall be called before God when we die. "Tyre and Sidon, Sodom and Gomorrah, Ninevah all will be called back. At the end of the world the Son of Man shall come and separate the wheat from the chaff" (Matt. 25). Augustine saw this life as a powerful sifting, grinding, and dividing experience. History was a millstone that was turning relentlessly, separating, selecting, crushing, cleaning. As heirs of the human story, we are subject to death and its judgment.

> We must confess, then, that had not our first parents sinned, they had not died: but sinning, the punishment of death was inflicted upon them and all of their posterity. . . . That which was penal in the first man's offending was made natural in the birth of all the rest. The dust was man's (Adam's) parents: but man is man's parent. (*C.D.* 13.3)

Augustine's summary of biblical teaching on life and death has exerted an inestimable influence on the course of history. If death is divine judgment on biological life, then it is in the death of the body that the deepest conflict about the nature and destiny of our existence will take place. It is in the realm of biological inheritance, in genetic transfer, in the congealing of human germinal cells, and in the developing human person that sin and death and grace and life are found in profound conflict. The plight of this body—its growth and development, its vitality and disorder, its energy and its demise—is the arena of the drama of guilt, grace, and redemption. Death itself, and dying as the call to death's journey (*Winterreise*), is the moment of God's ultimate conflict with us and through us with adversarial power. Our death, then, is the final battlefield where Christ's resurrection is verified in nature.

A brief excursus on the juridical, biomedical, pastoral, and theological significance of an Augustinian Reformed ethics of dying and death can now be suggested.

First, in the case of criminal justice, even if the accused pleads culpability and asks for death (e.g., Gary Gilmore), the state should be very reluctant to use this power. In the same way, the physician should not aid a patient who in overwhelming suffering pleads for death. In the same way, a person should not consider suicide as a course to relieve anguish. In all of these cases life is being cut short and the redemptive enactment of the soul's struggle is foreshortened: it "leaves no place in the soul for saving repentance" (*C.D.* 1.16.17). The juridical impact of these beliefs on questions of capital punishment, euthanasia, and suicide is far-reaching. We are to stand back in awe, respect, and care before a person's dying. In his self, the cosmic struggle of death and resurrection is being enacted. We must arrogate that hastening and delaying power to ourselves only in rare circumstances.

Second, biomedically speaking, the Reformed doctrine of death, judgment, and resurrection has framed the basic tension between saving and prolonging life, on the one hand, and not inflicting death or perpetuating dying, on the other. Why do we fight to save life? While it is in part motivated by our moral abhorrence of idly watching someone die while we could prevent it, the deeper impulse is to allow more life, more redemptive possibility, for the soul. When the conquistadores baptized pagan children and then smashed their heads on rocks to save them from the damning possibilities of continuing life, they may have appealed to Augustine, certainly in his late magisterial work (the indelible grace of the church's sacraments), but they were in violent opposition to the direction of his ethic. Death is an appointment with destiny. Our responsible role is to watch near with care and succor, restraining ourselves from coercing or retarding its enactment.

Third, the pastoral implication of this doctrine is to exhort us to live as if preparing to die and to attend one another with reverence in the process of dying. Since this is the grand culmination of life and the preparation to meet God, the dying person has profound wisdom to impart. If spared the indignities of officious management and thoughtless neglect, if allowed the grace (perhaps by medicine) of clear mind and speech, the dying one is our best teacher about living. The deathbed scene of ages past, when the family was summoned to receive blessing, forgiveness, and counsel, has been abandoned to our great impoverishment. Even when pain or disease renders one mute or incapacitated, one's courage and character disclosed in death leave their mark on all who participate. There is no greater sermon than that given by one who dies in Christ.

Fourth, the theological spirit of Augustine as sustained through Anselm (eleventh century) to Calvin does not exult in the damnation of sinners or in the death-boundedness of all of us because of the Fall. Calvin simply says with gentle humility that Christ's obedience has made us righteous and alive before God, just as Adam's disobedience had brought disgrace and death to the whole human family (Rom. 5:18). The solidarity of the whole human race is a fundamental belief for Calvin. Just as the first Adam incurred guilt and the second secured grace for humankind, so our actions have impact on the species itself. To kill a man is to assault the entire human community (one wishes that Calvin had remembered this the Sunday morning Servetus wandered into Geneva). To bring life is to grace the entire family. The high responsibility of vocation and the achievement of good is understood from this perspective.

The commandment "not to kill" is the commandment to give, sustain, and enhance life. When Thomas Sydenham was trained in Calvin's theology by his Puritan parents or when, at Princeton, Presbyterian President Witherspoon instructed James Madison in the Calvinist doctrine that would shape the American Constitution, the emphasis was on secular-humanistic work as our repudiation of death in the name of Christ's redemptive life (*Institutes*, 2.7.6, p. 404).

Finally, Calvin counseled against the mania to know the facts and details of pre- or post-death existence. The fascination with the topography of heaven, hell, and limbo or with the *via dolorosa* of the stages of dying is offensive to the Reformed spirit:

> Let us be content with the limits divinely set for us . . . the souls of the pious, having ended the toil for their warfare, enter into blessed rest, where in glad expectation they await the promised glory . . . until Christ the redeemer appear. (*Institutes*, 3.25, p. 998)

The Puritan spirit took the secular side of Calvin's eschatology and awaited redemption of this body and the return of Christ to this history in the impending future. Puritans indeed felt that the earthly kingdom was starting to appear in universal history (explorers had circumnavigated the globe), in communication (the printing press and universal commerce had appeared), and in the dawn of empirical science (not thwarted by debilitating Aristotelian theory, new explorations of the body and mind were opening new truth). The Puritans believed, quite in the spirit of Augustine and Calvin, that sin and death manifested themselves in our physical body. Therefore, aging and the corruption of disease were consequences of the Fall. What do we do? Do we attempt to overcome the Fall? Do we seek to liberate childbirth from its anguish and daily work from its toil? No! These are the enduring and irremovable results of our primal transgression. What we must do is seek to open up the greatest spiritual freedom in our existence (through learning, piety, science) in order that the physical manifestations of spiritual renewal might be more manifest. God is slowly but perceptibly redeeming this world of his through the agency of his creaturely likeness, human beings. If their sin—avarice, exploitation, destructiveness—can be restrained and if creative knowledge and technology can flourish again in this despoiled creation, the age of Christ will begin to dawn. Jonathan Edwards and the American Puritans saw it coming: the plagues were waning, temperance and social justice were flourishing in the Great Awakening, smallpox vaccination was working—Christ was making vigorous assault on Satan's strongholds.

In the centuries from the Puritan age to ours we have pursued the millenarian vision, particularly in its technical and political senses, but we have abandoned the underlying theological rationale. Today we find ourselves supporting a scientific culture that assaults death, and we don't know why. We find ourselves drawn to Eastern and primitive world views that see nature as static or cyclic because we fear the intensity of the scientific and biological revolution, we are suspicious of the men who move it, and we are not sure where it will lead. The only way our nerve (as well as appropriate scientific goals) can be restored is to recover the spiritual roots of the enterprise. In the eighteenth and nineteenth centuries we vacillated between a romantic materialism, on the one hand, that moved in defiance of God and human value to establish unbridled human technical power over life and, on the other hand, a rigid theological formalism or otherworldly pietism that despaired of anything fruitful arising in the human project. What we need is a renewed vision of the human prospect under God. In life and death this means: a sense of amazement and gratitude for life in its natural goodness and natural boundaries and a commitment to secure the fullness of that possibility for all. Second, it means a vision of the redeemed humanity and world that Christ is creating, with a healthy appreciation of human frailty and a critical stance toward human ambitions and goals along with a commitment to a better world in which evil and necessity are not accepted but death is viewed as a challenge—God's opportunity with us. Third, this renewed vision means a view of human solidarity whereby the blessings of knowledge, technology, healing power, and the like are shared with all and the kingdom of evil is thereby diminished.

The Reformed doctrine of death and resurrection can be summarized in this way: drawn in ecstasy into God's redemption we are given entrance into this life with new verve and vitality. We celebrate life just as we welcome death, for Christ has met us at the boundary. G. C. Berkouwer has summarized Karl Barth's rich reflection on this theme:

> God permits nothing to be lost—no hue in deepest ocean depths, no wing-beat of an insect that lives but a day, not the earliest time in earth's history, and certainly nothing in our life. God will not be alone in His eternity, but He will be together with His creature, His creature in its limited duration. "Present before God—this way the creature will be and will remain" (*Dogmatics*, III/2, pp. 102–103). This is the way in which it will be enfolded in the great rest of God.[31]

Case Study: Dying into Life

She lay under the oxygen tent: a young woman with young children. She was a nurse in the best tradition, one who knew the terrors patients faced in their last hours. She also knew the peace they experienced. Now she herself lay dying with a fulminating leukemia that took only weeks to seize her life. Through the misty plastic tent she could see me standing nervously, wondering what I should say or do. She was a good friend and I was scared —for her, for me, for her husband, for her family. She beckoned with her hand. I zipped open the tent and leaned in. She looked up and smiled, "What are you worried about?" In death she gave life in the name of her Lord who had done the same for her.

Postscript

After all the expositions of Reformed doctrines have been laid aside, the enduring tradition is borne along in the lives of those men and women, boys and girls, whose belief, hope, and capacity to care have been nurtured by that faith community. The tradition is thus perpetually being remade in the mind and heart of each person who is drawn through that community to the person-event that lies at the center of history—the life, death, resurrection, and everliving presence of Jesus Christ. His holy spirit is the Lord, the giver of life. Our transactions of life's crises of health and disease and our unending quest to make sense of life's bliss and vicissitudes gravitate to this center. The tradition becomes a composite phenomenon as common faith is expressed across the continents and across the ages. I discover my own roots as I meet friends of German Reformed faith from the Rhineland or Calvinist theologians from Strasbourg, France.

Throughout this text we have repeatedly called on the insights of Shakespeare, a writer who truly transcends all traditions. Mahatma Gandhi, another universal man, read the Hindu scriptures, prayed Muhammed's prayers, and sang Christ's hymns. In our time a similarly ecumenical tradition is being formed, wherein Hindu, Jew, and Muslim remind us of the lost treasure in our Christian tradition, thereby calling us to that grand tradition (yet to be formed) that alone can guide us into this age of universal history. The themes of life and health, of suffering and death, may provide windows to glimpse that promised future wherein we shall all be one, and peace and health shall reign on earth.

Notes

Preface

   1. Karl Barth, *Ethics* (Edinburgh: T & T. Clark, 1981); idem, *The Knowledge of God and the Service of God* (London: Hodder and Stoughton, 1938), Barth's 1937–1938 Gifford Lectures based on the Scots Confession of 1560, a major sixteenth-century Reformed document.

Introduction: Definitions

   1. Alasdair MacIntyre, *After Virtue* (London: Duckworth, 1981), p. 119.
   2. Ibid., p. 202.
   3. Gordon Rupp, *Six Makers of English Religion 1500–1700* (London: Hodder and Stoughton, 1957), p. x.
   4. MacIntyre, p. 137.
   5. Arnold Toynbee, *Mankind and Mother Earth: A Narrative History of the World* (Oxford: Oxford University Press, 1976), p. 536.
   6. Max Weber, *The Protestant Ethic and the Spirit of Capitalism* (London, 1930); R. H. Tawney, *Religion and the Rise of Capitalism* (New York, 1927).
   7. V. H. H. Green, *Luther and the Reformation* (London: B. T. Batsford, 1964), p. 13; see also pp. 11–26.
   8. On Calvin and Servetus, see James K. Cameron, "Scottish Calvinism and the Principle of Intolerance," in *Reformatio Perennis*, ed. B. A. Gerrish, with Robert Benedetto (Pittsburgh: Pickwick Press, 1981). On Cromwell, see Christopher Hill, *The World Turned Upside Down* (New York: Penguin Books, 1975).
   Thanks to Donald Norwood, Oxford, for help in this and other matters of Reformed doctrine.

Part I/WHAT DO WE BELIEVE? THE NATURE OF GOD

   1. For an overview of modern mainline Presbyterian belief, see John McKay, *The Presbyterian Way of Life* (Englewood Cliffs, N.J.: Prentice-Hall, 1960).
   2. John Calvin, *The Institutes of the Christian Religion*, 2 vols., ed. John T. McNeill, Library of Christian Classics, vols. 20 and 21 (Philadelphia: Westminster, 1960); hereafter cited as *Institutes*.

Chapter 1/The Reformed Tradition: Beliefs and Questions

   1. *The Scots Confession of 1560* (Edinburgh: Saint Andrew Press), p. 33; hereafter cited as Scots Confession.
   2. Melito of Sardis, *Homily on the Passion*, par. II, ed. C. Bonner (Philadelphia: Penn Press, 1940), p. 168.
   3. Paul Tillich, *A History of Christian Thought* (London: SCM Press, 1968), p. 231.
   4. C. F. D. Moule, *The Origin of Christology* (Cambridge: Cambridge University Press, 1977), p. 143.
   5. Romanum, *Old Roman Baptismal Creed* (early second century). See H. Leitzmann, *The Founding of the Church Universal* (London: Lutterworth, 1938), p. 143.
   6. Paul Tillich, "Science and Theology: A Discussion with Einstein," *Theology of Culture* (New York: Oxford University Press, 1959) pp. 127ff.

7. Augustine, *Civitas Dei* 19.3; hereafter cited as *C.D.* and quoted from the edition of J. L. Vives (London, 1620).

8. The Confession of 1967 of the Presbyterian Church, for instance, focused on reconciliation.

9. P. Lain Entralgo, *The Therapy of the Word in Classical Antiquity* (New Haven: Yale University Press, 1970).

10. John Hick, *The Center of Christianity* (London: SCM Press, 1977), p. 106.

11. L. Berkhof, *Systematic Theology* (Grand Rapids: Eerdmans, 1939), pp. 265ff.

12. Cf. Jürgen Moltmann, *The Crucified God* (London: SCM Press, 1973); and Daniel Day Williams, "Suffering and Being in Empirical Theology," in *The Future of Empirical Theology*, ed. Bernard E. Meland (Chicago: University of Chicago Press, 1969).

13. H. Richard Niebuhr, *Christ and Culture* (London: Faber and Faber, 1952), pp. 217–18.

Part II/HOW SHALL WE ACT? HUMAN LIFE

Chapter 2/Being Human: Life's Powers and Predicaments

1. See Constitution of the World Health Organization (1946), in *Official Records of the World Health Organization*, 2:100.

2. F. D. Maurice, *Conflict of Good and Evil in Our Day* (London: Smith, Elder and Co., 1865), p. 27.

3. See Wallace E. Anderson, ed., *The Works of Jonathan Edwards: Scientific and Philosophical Writings* (New Haven: Yale University Press, 1980).

4. Robert Boyle, *A Disquisition About the Final Causes of Natural Things* (London, 1688), pp. 22–23.

5. Isaac Newton, *Optics* (1706 edition), Query 31, p. 348.

6. Friedrich Schleiermacher, *On Religion: Speeches to Its Cultured Despisers*, trans. John Oman (New York: Harper Bros., 1958), p. 100.

7. Maurice, pp. 15–17.

8. George Bernard Shaw, "Preface to the Doctor's Dilemma," in *Prefaces* (London: Odhams, 1938), p. 280.

9. "U.S. Approves Selling of New Human Insulin," *International Herald Tribune*, October 30, 1982, p. 3.

10. C. S. Lewis, *The Abolition of Man* (New York: Macmillan, 1965), p. 71.

11. *"Psychē,"* in Gerhard Kittel and Gerhard Friedrich, eds., *Theological Dictionary of the New Testament*, vol. 9 (Grand Rapids: Eerdmans, 1973), pp. 608ff.

12. Ibid., pp. 626–27.

13. Augustine, *On Exodus*, 21. 80, Corpus Scriptorum Ecclesiasticorum Latinorum (Vienna, 1866), 28.2.147.

14. Karl Barth, *The Epistle to the Romans* (Oxford: Oxford University Press, 1933); *From Rousseau to Ritschl* (London: SCM Press, 1959).

15. See David Cox, *Jung and St. Paul* (London: Longmans, Green and Co., 1959), p. 30.

16. Stanley Hauerwas, *Truthfulness and Tragedy* (Notre Dame: University of Notre Dame Press, 1977), pp. 127ff.

17. See Paul Ramsey, *The Patient as Person* (New Haven: Yale University Press, 1978).

18. C. S. Lewis, *The Problem of Pain* (London: Centenary Press, 1940).

19. Ibid., p. 77.

20. Victor Fuchs, *Who Shall Live? Health, Economics, and Social Change* (New York: Basic Books, 1974), p. 53. However, it must be noted that the Mormons suffer more from neurological and prostate tumors than does the general populace.

21. See Eric Osborn, *Ethical Patterns in Early Christian Thought* (Cambridge: Cambridge University Press, 1976), p. 35.

22. See John Bowker, *Problems of Suffering in Religions of the World* (Cambridge: Cambridge University Press, 1970), pp. 86ff.

23. Augustine, "Sermon on Psalm 137," *Expositions on the Book of Psalms* (Oxford: Parker, 1857), p. 162.

24. See Henry Adams, *Mont-St.-Michel and Chartres* (1913).

25. See Paul Tillich, *A History of Christian Thought* (London: SCM Press, 1968), pp. 266–67.

26. T. H. L. Parker, ed., *Calvin's Sermons on Isaiah 53* (London: James Clark, 1956), p. 64.

27. Mark Zborowski, *People in Pain* (New York: Jossey-Bass, 1968).

28. Maurice, *Conflict of Good and Evil*, p. 29.

29. H. Richard Niebuhr, *The Responsible Self* (New York: Harper and Row, 1963), p. 59.

30. James Gustafson, *Theology and Ethics* (Oxford: Basil Blackwell, 1981), p. 249.

31. William McNeill, *Plagues and Peoples* (New York: Simon and Schuster, 1978), p. 282.

32. Jürgen Moltmann, *The Theology of Hope* (New York: Harper and Row, 1964), p. 25.

33. Pierre Teilhard de Chardin, *Hymn to the Universe* (London: Collins, 1965), p. 20.

34. In reality, if Mani, Augustine, and Pelagius met today, the close affinity of their views might lead them to form church together. Pelagius, in fact, although he has been labeled the advocate of "human initiative in salvation," wrote the first important treatise on *sola fide, sola gratia*.

35. Augustine, "On the Proceedings of Pelagius," *The Nicene and Post-Nicene Fathers*, vol. 5 (Grand Rapids: Eerdmans, 1956), p. 192.

36. Erik Erikson, *Young Man Luther* (London: Faber, 1958), pp. 198–200.

37. See Rudolf Hermann, *Luthers These "Girecht und Sunde zugleich"* (Berlin: Gutersloh, 1930).

38. John Calvin, *Commentaries: Romans and Thessalonians I, II* (London: Oliver and Boyd, 1961), pp. 148ff.

39. Barth, *The Epistle to the Romans*, p. 259.

40. Ibid., p. 260.

41. Robert Burton, as quoted in "Melancholy," in J. Hastings, ed., *Encyclopedia of Religion and Ethics*, vol. 8 (Edinburgh: T. & T. Clark, 1915), pp. 526ff.

42. William James, *The Varieties of Religious Experience* (London: Longmans, Green and Co., 1937), pp. 163–64.

43. See *The Martin Luther Christmas Book*, trans. and arranged by Roland Bainton (Philadelphia: Muhlenberg Press, 1948).

44. R. D. Laing, *The Politics of Experience* (Harmondsworth: Penguin Books, 1964), p. 63.

45. Ibid., p.3.

46. See Thomas Szass, *The Theology of Medicine* (Oxford: Oxford University Press, 1979), pp. 126ff.

47. Karl Menninger, *The Crime of Punishment* (New York: Viking Press, 1968), pp. 260–61.

48. See Edgar Z. Friedenberg, *Laing* (London: Woburn Press, 1974), p. 20.

49. Ibid., p. 18.

50. Flannery O'Connor, *A Good Man Is Hard to Find* (London: Women's Press, 1980), pp. 52ff.

Chapter 3/Becoming Human: Life's Transitions and Transactions

1. Quotations from *As You Like It* are taken from the New Clarendon Shakespeare (Oxford: At the Clarendon Press, 1962).

2. Erik Erikson, *Young Man Luther* (London: Faber and Faber, 1958), p. 247. Erikson's master framework is developed in *Childhood and Society* (New York: Norton, 1950).

3. *Young Man Luther*, pp. 248–49.

4. Ibid., pp. 245ff.

5. See *Childhood and Society*, passim.

6. *Pensées*; see L. C. Brunschvicg, *Blaise Pascal, Opuscules et Pensées* (Paris, 1897), p. 80.

7. See Reinhold Niebuhr, *Beyond Tragedy* (London: Nisbet and Co., 1938); and John Baillie, *The Belief in Progress* (Oxford: Oxford University Press, 1950).

8. "Hesiod," in J. Hastings, ed., *Encyclopedia of Religion and Ethics*, vol. 6 (Edinburg: T. & T. Clark, 1913), pp. 668ff.

9. Wolfhart Pannenberg, *Ethics* (London: Search Press, 1981), p. 9.

10. See Peter Brown, *Augustine of Hippo* (London: Faber and Faber, 1967), p. 403.

11. All quotes to the Westminster Confession are from John H. Leith, *Creeds of All Churches* (New York: Anchor Books, 1963). Here see p. 197.

12. See Otto Beall, *Cotton Mather: The First Significant Figure in American Medicine* (Baltimore: Johns Hopkins Press, 1969).

13. See Paul Tillich, *Perspective on Nineteenth and Twentieth Century Protestant Theology* (London: SCM Press, 1967), p. 111.

14. *The Observer*'s article was based on research reported by Dr. Alayne Yates and colleagues, of the University of Arizona Health Sciences Center, in the *New England Journal of Medicine*.

15. Ivan Illich, *Limits to Medicine* (London: Marion Boyars, 1976), pp. 204–5.

16. Philip Schaff, *The Teaching of the Twelve Apostles (Didache)* (New York: Funk and Wagnalls, 1890), p. 169.

17. See John T. Noonan, Jr., ed., *The Morality of Abortion: Legal and Historical Perspectives* (Cambridge: Harvard University Press, 1972), pp. 4ff.

18. Samuel Laeuchli, *Power and Sexuality: The Emergence of Canon Law at the Synod of Elvira* (Philadelphia: Temple University Press, 1972), p. 130.

19. Thomas Sydenham, *Opera Omnia*, ed. Guiliemus Alexander Greenhill, M. D. (London: Impensis Societatis Sydenhamianae, 1844), Preface, p. 14.

20. Friedrich Schleiermacher, *On Religion*, p. 131.

21. F. D. Maurice, *Social Morality* (London: Macmillan and Co., 1872), pp. 44–45.

22. See James Gustafson, *Theology and Ethics* (Chicago: University of Chicago Press, 1981); see also Gustafson's other writings such as *Theology and Medical Ethics*. See also Kenneth Vaux, *Biomedical Ethics* (New York: Harper and Row, 1974).

23. Schubert Ogden, *Faith and Freedom: Toward a Theology of Liberation* (Nashville: Abingdon, 1978), p. 37.

24. Baruch Brody, *Abortion and the Sanctity of Human Life* (Boston: MIT Press, 1975), p. 2.

25. John Locke, "Vindication of the Reasonableness of Christianity," in *Works*, vol. 7 (London, 1823), p. 178.

26. John Calvin, "Commentary on John" (1:5), in *Opera*, XLVII 6 d; cf. 1:9 (9b), Corpus Reformatorum, ed. H. W. Baum et al. (Brunswick: Schwetschke, 1863–1900).

27. See Edward A. Dowey, Jr., *The Knowledge of God in Calvin's Theology* (New York: Columbia University Press, 1952), pp. 15ff.

Chapter 4/Acting Human: Life's Choices and Destiny

1. Paul Lehmann, *Ethics in a Christian Context* (London: SCM Press, 1963), p. 25. Lehmann quotes in this chapter come from this source.

2. Jeremy Taylor, *The Rule and Exercizes of Holy Living and Holy Dying* (1650–51), The Ancient and Modern Library of Theological Literature (London: Griffith, Farran, Okeden and Welsh).

3. Karl Barth, *The Epistle to the Romans* (Oxford: Oxford University Press, 1933), p. 425.

4. See Joseph Fletcher, *Medicine and Morals* (Princeton: Princeton University Press, 1954).

5. Gerald Dworkin, "Paternalism," *The Monist* 56, no. 1 (1972): 64–84. A larger study on autonomy is as yet unpublished.

6. Plato, quoted in Eric Osborn, *Ethical Pattern in Early Christian Thought* (Cambridge: Cambridge University Press, 1967), p. 7.

8. Rudolf Bultmann, *Theology of the New Testament* vol. 2, (London: Routledge, 1955), p. 226.

8. William Tyndale, *Expositions* (London: Parker Society, 1853), p. 6.

9. William Tyndale, *Doctrinal Treatises* 7 (London: Parker Society, 1853).

10. See Paul Tillich, *A History of Christian Thought* (London: SCM Press, 1968), pp. 288–89.

11. Lionel Tiger and Robin Fox, *The Imperial Animal* (London: Secker and Warburg, 1972), pp. 240–41.

12. Leslie Weatherhead, "Present-day Non-Medical Method of Healing," in *Religion and Medicine*, ed. John Crowleysmith (London: Epworth Press, 1962), p. 32.

13. Paul Tillich, "Heal the Sick, Cast out Demons," *The Eternal Now* (London: SCM Press, 1963), pp. 47ff.; page numbers in this section refer to this printing of the sermon.

14. See Otto Beall, *Cotton Mather; The First Significant Figure in American Medicine* (Baltimore: John Hopkins Press, 1969).

15. Origin, *Contra Celsum* 1.24.25; French edition, *Contre Celse*, v. 132, livres 1–11 (Paris: Du Cerf, 1967), pp. 135ff.

16. Paul Ramsey, "The Nature of Medical Ethics," in *Ethics in Medicine*, ed. A. Dyck and S. Reiser (Cambridge: MIT Press, 1977), p. 128. See also Ramsey's *The Patient as Person* (New Haven: Yale University Press, 1970).

17. Norman Cohn, *The Pursuit of the Millennium* (New York: Harper and Row, 1961), p. 201.

18. John Wycliffe, *De civilo domino*, in *Wyclif's Latin Works*, ed. Reginald Poole, vol. 1, (London: Wyclif Society, 1895), chap. xiv, p. 96H.

19. Martin Luther, *The Freedom of a Christian*, in *Luther's Works*, vol. 31, ed. Harold J. Grimm (Philadelphia: Muhlenberg Press, 1957), p. 344.

20. I am indebted for this insight to Oliver O'Donovan, Regius Professor of Moral Theology at Christ Church Oxford. See his *The Concept of Self-Love in Augustine* (New Haven: Yale University Press, 1981).

21. Gustavo Gutierrez, "Faith and Freedom Are Living with Change," in *Experience and Faith*, ed. Francis Eigo (Villanova, Penn.: Villanova University Press, 1976), p. 25.

22. Ogden, p. 93.

23. Gutierrez, p. 25.

24. See James Childress, *Priorities in Biomedical Ethics* (Philadelphia: Westminster Press, 1983), pp. 76ff.

25. Charles Dickens, *Dombey and Son* (1848).

26. Anthony Trollope, *Barchester Towers* (1857).

27. On this subject, see Kenneth Vaux, *Will to Live, Will to Die* (Minneapolis: Augsburg Press, 1978).

28. John Bunyan, *The Pilgrim's Progress* (London: Ernest Wister, 1678), pp. 345–46.

29. Gilgamesh Epic, tablet 1, iii, 3–4, Anet 90, quoted in "Death," George A. Buttrick and Keith R. Crim, eds., *The Interpreter's Dictionary of the Bible*, vol. 1 (Nashville: Abingdon, 1962), p. 803.

30. E. B. Pusey, quoted in John Hick, *The Center of Christianity*, (London: SCM Press, 1977), p. 200.

31. G. C. Berkouwer, *The Triumph of Grace in the Theology of Karl Barth* (London: Patternoster, 1956), p. 164.